The image above shows a SPECT scan of my brain during SVT, with increased blood flow and activity in the prefrontal cortex and basal ganglia. This EEG (below) shows my brainwaves on SVT, with an overall increase in theta brain waves and a large boost of beta brain waves in the occipital lobe. See page 35 for complete results.

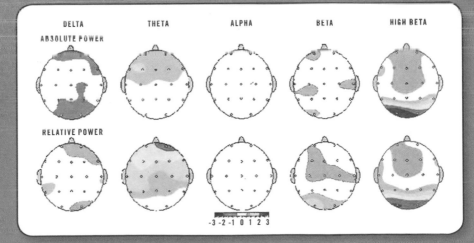

—— YOUR ——

SUBCONSCIOUS

—— BRAIN CAN ——

CHANGE YOUR LIFE

ALSO BY DR. MIKE DOW

Chicken Soup for the Soul: Think, Act, & Be Happy:
How to Use Chicken Soup for the Soul Stories to
Train Your Brain to Be Your Own Therapist

Heal Your Drained Brain: Naturally Relieve Anxiety, Combat
Insomnia, and Balance Your Brain in Just 14 Days

Healing the Broken Brain: Leading Experts
Answer 100 Questions about Stroke Recovery

The Brain Fog Fix: Reclaim Your Focus,
Memory, and Joy in Just 3 Weeks

All of the above are available at your local bookstore,
or may be ordered by visiting:

Hay House USA: www.hayhouse.com®
Hay House Australia: www.hayhouse.com.au
Hay House UK: www.hayhouse.co.uk
Hay House India: www.hayhouse.co.in

* * *

YOUR
SUBCONSCIOUS
BRAIN CAN
CHANGE YOUR LIFE

Overcome Obstacles,
Heal Your Body, and Reach Any Goal
with a Revolutionary Technique

DR. MIKE DOW

HAY HOUSE, INC.
Carlsbad, California • New York City
London • Sydney • New Delhi

Published in the United States by: Hay House, Inc.: www.hayhouse.com®
Published in Australia by: Hay House Australia Pty. Ltd.: www.hayhouse.com.au
Published in the United Kingdom by: Hay House UK, Ltd.: www.hayhouse.co.uk
Published in India by: Hay House Publishers India: www.hayhouse.co.in

Cover design: Ploy Siripant • *Interior design:* Joe Bernier
Indexer: Joan D. Shapiro

Cataloging-in-Publication Data is on file at the Library of Congress

Hardcover ISBN: 978-1-4019-5585-4
E-book ISBN: 978-1-4019-5586-1

10 9 8 7 6 5 4 3 2 1
1st edition, March 2019

Printed in the United States of America

SUSTAINABLE
FORESTRY
INITIATIVE
Certified Chain of Custody
Promoting Sustainable Forestry
www.sfiprogram.org
SFI-01268

SFI label applies to the text stock

CONTENTS

Foreword by Dr. Daniel Amen ix

Introduction: Subconscious Visualization Technique:
The Ultimate Mindbody Medicine xiii

PART I: Understanding Your Subconscious

Chapter 1: Your Subconscious Always Has Your Back 3

Chapter 2: The Science of the Subconscious Brain 21

Chapter 3: A Conscious Start to Subconscious Healing: SVT Step 1 . . .41

Chapter 4: Activating the Subconscious Brain: SVT Step 2 51

Chapter 5: Seamless SVT: Adding Steps 3 Through 7 65

Chapter 6: Power Boost SVT 73

PART II: Putting SVT to Work for You

Chapter 7: SVT for Letting Go 87

Chapter 8: SVT to Stress Less and Conquer Fears 111

Chapter 9: SVT to Boost Your Mood 137

Chapter 10: SVT for Habits and Healthier Living 161

Chapter 11: SVT for Healing Your Body, Pain,
and Elusive Conditions 183

Appendix A: Bonus SVT Practice for Sleep, Insomnia,
and Induced Dreaming 223

Appendix B: Bonus SVT Practice for Success 231

Appendix C: Bonus SVT Practice for Spiritual Connection 236

Appendix D: SVT Downloads 242

Endnotes 244

Index 255

About the Author 263

FOREWORD

Your brain shifts between the conscious and the subconscious all the time. The most obvious transition is when you fall asleep and dream. The shift also occurs throughout the day. When you go to the theater and a two-hour movie feels like it's over in a half hour—that's your subconscious brain at work. Or consider a long road trip: when I drove from Southern California to Oklahoma for medical school, I couldn't remember driving through several cities on the route—that's called highway hypnosis. My mind was on "autopilot."

After a 40-year career as a psychiatrist, brain-imaging expert, founder of the Amen Clinics, and creator of brain-health programs around the world, I know a lot about the brain. At the Amen Clinics, we've been looking at the brain for over 25 years. You could say I'm always in someone's head!

The brain is a symphony of parts that work together to create and sustain a life. Yet most people don't think about their brains, much less the subconscious part of it. The subconscious is amazing and can do a great deal to create health and transformation between your brain and body.

Would you like to know how?

I certainly did.

I first became interested in the power of the subconscious brain when I was a second-year med student. One of my professors hypnotized a few of his students, placing them into a subconscious-dominant state. When he used the technique on me, I felt more peaceful than ever before. I quickly learned that hypnosis doesn't tune you out; it tunes you in.

Soon afterward, I took a one-month elective on hypnosis at the University of California, Irvine. My professor there showed us a video of an Indian psychiatrist who guided a patient into a hypnotic state and then used her subconscious brain to make the blood vessels pop up in her hands so he could insert a needle. It worked—and I was fascinated. So during my first rotation as an intern in the emergency room at Walter Reed Army Medical Center in Washington, D.C., I got the bright idea to try the technique myself.

At 6:30 A.M., I walked by a room where a woman was screaming. Since I'm super curious, I popped in. The woman had a blood clot in her calf that was causing her leg to swell. The chief resident was screaming at the patient because every time she tried to start the IV needle, the patient screamed louder. So the chief resident was frustrated, and the patient was scared. And guess what happens to blood vessels when you're upset—they clamp down! So I asked the chief resident, "Do you mind if I try?"

"I've been starting IVs for years. What makes you think you can do it?" she replied. "But if you want to try, hotshot, go ahead."

The first thing I did was say to the patient, "Hi, I'm Dr. Amen. I need you to slow your breathing. When you breathe too fast, all your blood vessels constrict, and there's no way we're going to start an IV on your foot. So breathe with me."

I slowed my own breathing to show her how, all while thinking, *The chief resident is going to kill me when this fails*—because I had no expectation this approach was going to work. But I'd just seen the video in my elective class. So I asked the patient to focus on a spot on the wall to help remove all the distractions. I guided her to count to ten, close her eyes, breathe slowly, and then imagine relaxation. While I was taking her through this process, I told her, "I bet you didn't know that if you focused on your feet, you could actually make a blood vessel appear and help me out in this situation." A blood vessel popped up as soon as I made the suggestion, and I was able to start the IV. The chief resident's mouth just dropped open.

That's when I got hooked on using the power of the subconscious brain to help people.

One of the first lessons in medical school was to do no harm and use the least toxic solution. If we could heal with words and without pills, how wonderful would that be? That's what surgeons, ob-gyns, dentists, psychiatrists, and therapists have been doing for decades. In this book, Dr. Mike Dow will show you how to do the same as a supplemental way to create health, break or build habits, boost your confidence or success, alleviate anxiety and fear, and so much more. I've seen subconscious brain techniques help people stop smoking, achieve and maintain a healthy weight, conquer insomnia, and relieve pain syndromes.

Later in my internship at Walter Reed, patients often came to me about sleeping problems and asked for sleeping pills. "Sure, I'll prescribe you a sleeping pill," I would say, "but first, can I hypnotize you to see if you really need it?" Every patient said yes, and because hypnosis activates the healing power of the subconscious, I only prescribed sleeping pills for half of those patients.

Most people don't realize that your body responds to every single thought you have. If you have negative thoughts, your hands get colder and wetter, your muscles tense, your heart rate variability goes down, and so forth. So if you tap into your subconscious, you can plant messages of health and transformation that your brain will then carry out for you. Wouldn't you like to tap into your subconscious brain? It's easy, painless, and effortless.

Dr. Mike Dow has been using subconscious brain activation techniques with his patients for years. And he visited my office recently so we could scan his brain in conscious and subconscious states. The results, which you'll read about, reveal the science behind the amazing power of the brain.

Ultimately, the goal of this book is to get you to be in charge of your own brain, and use your subconscious to change your life.

—Daniel G. Amen, M.D.
Psychiatrist, neuroscientist, and founder of Amen Clinics
Author of *Feel Better Fast and Make It Last*

INTRODUCTION

Subconscious Visualization Technique: The Ultimate Mindbody Medicine

This book is surprising. Its program is revolutionary. To some, it may even be controversial. But in the end, Subconscious Visualization Technique, which is the protocol you'll learn and use, can make you healthier, happier, and even wealthier. If you think the subconscious brain is some woo-woo pseudoscience, get ready to have your mind blown.

The groundbreaking research I'll share with you proves that tapping into the power of the subconscious brain is a "hard" science, not a Vegas sideshow. I'll begin by showing you how your subconscious has already been conspiring in your favor—even if you haven't realized it.

I'll help you understand the difference between the conscious and the subconscious brain. You'll learn the best times to use each one (which, scientifically speaking, is actually an activation of certain brain *structures* in the brain itself).

For example, you can activate the subconscious to heal your past, boost creativity, or hack your way into parts of yourself that are off limits to the conscious brain. Did you know you can even change the way you digest food or interpret thoughts via the subconscious? By doing so, the conscious can do what it does best: handle the everyday, ho-hum happenings of your daily life. Let this less mysterious part of your brain handle math and fill out applications. Invite the subconscious brain to conspire in your favor and weave creative dreams that could change your life—and the world.

For those of you who doubt the power of the subconscious, I'll show you just how potent it can be. I'll geek out in a chapter filled with published research, brain scans, EEGs, and a bunch of scientific mumbo jumbo. Better yet, I'll show you a scan of my own brain as I use something I call *Subconscious Visualization Technique*, or *SVT*. If you'd like to start using SVT right away, you can skip to Chapter 3 and begin using the protocol—but I hope you don't. Most people find all the brain science that I cover in the earlier chapters to be incredibly fascinating. I've even seen patients' conscious understanding of the subconscious allow SVT to work even better.

After the theoretical understanding of the subconscious brain is behind us, it will be time for the magic—or should I say science?—to begin. You'll be conducting your own revolutionary experiment. This time, the subject will be you. (A note: While SVT is very effective with children, the at-home SVT practice should only be used by adults.)

No matter what your goal may be, this book may very well be the missing puzzle piece you've been searching for. Perhaps you seek to heal that elusive condition or chronic pain or take your business to the next level.

What exactly is Subconscious Visualization Technique? It's a revolutionary protocol I created. You'll learn all about it in this book, and the audio tracks I've prepared for you to download (see page 242) will allow you to experience it in a visceral way. It's the first and only protocol to combine hypnosis with cognitive behavioral therapy (CBT), mindfulness, guided visualization, audio-visual entrainment, and bilateral stimulation (utilizing the left and right sides of the body to access both sides of the brain).

Don't worry if you have no idea what any of this clinical mumbo jumbo means. You don't need to. In fact, there's no need for you to understand what's happening for the magic (oops, I mean science) to work. SVT is about immersing yourself in the experience itself—to heal and enhance your life.

Would you be surprised to discover that SVT works more quickly than techniques that rely on conscious channels to heal or to help you reach your goals? It is also more powerful and can create fantastic transformation. Why? Several reasons.

First, SVT allows you access to memories that the conscious does not. As you'll learn in Chapter 2—the nerdy brain science chapter—this is thanks to slow theta brain waves. Theta brain waves have been proven to help you access forgotten memories, including memories you weren't consciously aware of. A childhood experience may have been holding you back from something in your relationships, health, or career. SVT allows you access to that file. SVT empowers you with the ability to edit and delete the memory file as well. What will it be like for you to take a journey in your mind's eye? Will it help you to express repressed feelings you've been bottling up for decades? When this happens, it can help your physical body to relax. Overactive parts in the emotional centers of your brain that prevent you from expressing yourself in your current relationship can be healed. For many people, this can change the way they act in their current relationships.

Second, SVT has the power to activate and enhance the incredible potential of mindbody healing. (I spell *mindbody* without a hyphen; you can't separate the interaction between mind and body.) If you find a surprising childhood memory and heal it, you may even find that physical symptoms and syndromes improve. Patients with irritable bowel syndrome (IBS) or painful bladder syndrome may notice pelvic tension even disappears. Wouldn't that be such a relief? Countless patients I have treated have been looking for these solutions all their lives, and SVT allows them to find the root of their ailments. If you find the root, you can heal it—instead of chronically medicating your symptoms.

Third, SVT activates the immune system by boosting T cells. This is helpful whether you are currently dealing with health conditions or would like to prevent them. The subconscious brain can do this far better than the conscious brain can. You see, your *conscious* has a tendency to focus on the *I-wonder-what-could-go-wrong-tomorrow* line of thought. Your *subconscious* tends to focus on the *I-wonder-what-I-could-create-tomorrow* thought train. It will be so captivating to find out what you'd like to focus your attention on.

When the conscious brain is busy worrying, stress hormones spike. That suppresses the immune system. New research shows that a malignant cell in one organ system is more likely to multiply and even spread to other parts of the body when the body is under stress.[1] But when the subconscious is busy weaving its magical dreams of abundance, creativity, and peace, stress hormones go down. The immune system is boosted. Did you know your mindbody has an inherent and natural healing system and that SVT activates it?

Some examples of these elusive syndromes that I use SVT to treat include fibromyalgia, chronic pain, autoimmune conditions, chronic fatigue syndrome, leaky gut, small intestinal bacterial overgrowth (SIBO), irritable bowel syndrome (IBS), migraines, painful bladder syndrome, anxiety disorders, and any other complex condition that prescription medications are minimally effective in treating, if they work at all.

SVT can be a great add-on to treatment for diseases that are directly linked to your immune system, such as cancer and HIV. In that scientific-mumbo-jumbo chapter I told you about, you'll read about an incredible study that looked at the way activating the subconscious increased T cells (a measure of your immune system's strength) in medical students at a prestigious research university.

Fourth, SVT can help you create abundance. Would you like to take your business to the next level? Is it time you finally turned your side hustle into a dream career? Is it time for you to start living with purpose and passion, not hijacked by fear? Do you want to attract the love of your life? Is this the year you'd like to say good-bye to your phobias? If your answer to any of these questions is yes, it's so nice to know that SVT can get you there.

There's a great line in the movie *The Field of Dreams*: "If you build it, he will come." SVT has a similar philosophy: if your subconscious brain can see it, your conscious brain can then create it.

Every time you do something, you change your brain. Did you know that? Simple, everyday, and seemingly insignificant choices like hopping on that treadmill or choosing broccoli over fries help create new pathways.

If your subconscious brain can see it, your conscious brain can then create it.

This is why I use some cognitive behavioral therapy (CBT) techniques to treat phobias, such as a fear of cats. I'd start by showing you a picture of a cat. Your *experience* of seeing a picture of a cat, and then eventually viewing an actual cat, tells the brain: "I did that!" And SVT supercharges CBT: your subconscious brain can create vivid experiences, even making you feel as though you are actually *holding* a cat. I have the brain scans to prove it: my own brain getting scanned while using SVT. Take a look at the color images on the insider front cover. Despite my eyes being closed, you'll see the visual part of my brain lighting up like a firecracker—just as though I were *seeing* and *experiencing* something. If you just take Xanax for your phobia, you're not providing the brain an experience that allows it to change. And you may be setting yourself up for addiction while slowing your brain down. Are you starting to see how SVT can help you get to the root of your problems—and transform them?

Subconscious activation tricks your brain into thinking it's already done something. This principle can be applied to anything you want to create, from building businesses to speaking in public to exercising more. SVT is guided visualization on steroids. It's so much more powerful than just "imagining." Get ready for Chapter 2—that nerdy science chapter—where a great study will show you just how magical this can be. And, of course, I'll show you a transformation worthy of one of those home remodeling shows: scans of my brain on a normal day and scans of my brain while using SVT.

Finally, SVT helps you access the best parts of yourself. In many ways, it helps you to tap into your true self: a human being who is inherently lovable with limitless potential. Did you know you have a unique set of gifts that were given to you to serve this world and others in a special way? Have you forgotten that? Some part of you knows this already, doesn't it?

Perhaps you've had some experience with hypnosis, dream analysis, guided imagery, music therapy, or another experience that taps into the subconscious and its signature slow theta brain waves. If so, I ask you to approach SVT with the wonder of a child encountering something for the first time. After all, picking something apart and analyzing it is a function of the conscious. Experiencing something and immersing yourself in it is where the subconscious can weave its scientifically proven spells.

I felt called to write this book because I believe the world needs SVT. And we need it now, right now. We live in a world where negativity, trauma, and chronic pain prevent people from remembering their inherent greatness. Too many people are trapped in the negative feedback loops of pain, depression, and self-doubt. These loops prevent them from offering their unique gifts and love to the world. Hormones and neurotransmitters are affected, which negatively affects behavior. This can actually lead to addiction to prescription pain medication and even cancer. I believe that too many people have forgotten their inherent goodness. If that's you, SVT can help restore you to your best, former self. I wonder if SVT will help you become an even *better* version of yourself than you have ever been.

We live in a world where negativity, trauma, and chronic pain prevent people from remembering their inherent greatness.

Let's do a mini-practice of SVT right now.

Can you remember a time in your life when you felt absolutely confident, happy, and free? What might your life be like if you could live in that space . . . or at least "hang out" there most of the time. Guess what? SVT can take you there. Yes. That's right. Right here and right now. Would you like to go?

This journey we're about to go on together is an exciting one. Now, perhaps you're beginning to understand what I mean when I say Your Subconscious Brain Can Change Your Life. *I mean it.*

I don't know why you picked up this book. But I have a feeling you know exactly what you'd like to change. And now, perhaps you're also feeling a little more hopeful about the potential for you to break through to that next level, remember your inherent goodness, and start an abundant life that serves others in a way that's unique to you. That's exciting, isn't it? Did you know that restoring purpose to your life helps to slow aging? Forget Botox. Use SVT instead, as it helps your immune system fight precancerous cells. And, of course, it will just help you feel better.

In a moment, I'm going to ask you to recite simple phrases to yourself. I ask that you use the childlike wonder, boundless optimism, and supreme faith of the subconscious brain with this exercise. If you notice a part of you saying, "That's not true," that's actually wonderful. You've identified the voice of the conscious! Keep your pulse on that voice.

If that voice pops up at any point in our journey together, turn the dial down on your conscious as we work to turn up the volume of the subconscious in its mission to deliver more happiness, hope, and healing to your life. I'll teach you how. Won't that be so wonderful? If you've picked up this book, I know that some deep part of you is hungry for this shift.

To officially start our journey together, here's the mini-exercise. I believe that some part of you knows that these phrases are inherently true.

Meditate on the following phrases, and let them wash over your brain and your body. For a moment, suspend your ordinary reality. If some part of you is still hesitant, just lean into it as an experiment to try it out. I wonder what your experience will give you. After all, your *experience is the ultimate wisdom, isn't it?*

As you recite the following words silently to yourself, perhaps you'll notice how you already know how to go "somewhere else." Do you notice relaxation somewhere in the body, or do you feel a sort of dreamy quality taking over the brain?

My mindbody knows how to heal itself.

My mindbody knows how to heal itself.

My mindbody knows how to heal itself.

Only I know what true health and happiness mean to me . . . and only I have the power to create it.

Only I know what true health and happiness mean to me . . . and only I have the power to create it.

Only I know what true health and happiness mean to me . . . and only I have the power to create it.

By starting your journey here, imagine the kind of health, healing, and abundance you will start manifesting for yourself.

Isn't it so nice to know that our healing has actually already begun?

Using This Book and Accompanying Audio Downloads

The first half of this book gives you the foundation for SVT and how it can empower you to change your behaviors, patterns, and thoughts. In the second half of the book, I take a deeper dive into the science of how SVT can be used to reach specific goals and the science supporting its use for groups of conditions. The second half of the book also contains the full SVT scripts, which are also offered to you as audio tracks (see page 242 for download information). Like meditation, SVT is a practice that can be used again and again. Its benefits multiply with repeated use. Most people will progress through the book and then use the SVT practice using the audio tracks once they reach the written scripts in this book. However, some people are so anxious to get started that they jump in with the audio tracks right away. If that's you, simply come back later to read the chapters on the details of what was happening to your brain. Either way, you'll probably find that you use each SVT audio track over and over again. And you'll probably find something useful in every audio track—even if that practice isn't your primary goal. While the steps of SVT are the same, each practice is unique.

In terms of using the audio tracks versus written scripts, I suggest using the corresponding audio tracks to begin SVT. This allows you to relax while I do the work of activating your subconscious brain and the power it has to heal and transform you. The audio tracks will also help you become familiar with SVT so that down the road, you'll be able to shift to a subconscious dominant state more quickly and activate your subconscious brain on your own at any time, any place. Later, you can come back and review the written scripts if you'd like to memorize SVT or become more proficient in it. To access the audio tracks, see page 242 or go to hayhouse .com/download and use the product code 5854 and the download code: Audio.

PART I

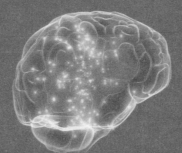

*Understanding
Your Subconscious*

CHAPTER 1

Your Subconscious Always Has Your Back

Whether you know it or not, you already use your subconscious brain all the time. Perhaps it took control of the wheel as your conscious mind was busy tackling a problem during a 30-minute drive home. You barely remember making your way home from the office, but somehow your car ended up safely in your driveway.

Perhaps a name escaped you during the day. Despite trying your hardest to remember it, the conscious parts of your brain couldn't retrieve what you were seeking. Then, your subconscious worked its magic and presented you with the answer hours later. That part of your brain had been hard at work for you all this time, and you didn't even realize it.

A similar phenomenon is at play when—all of a sudden—you remember how you knew someone after you gave up searching for the connection. Oh, that's right! He was your friend's husband; you met him at that dinner two years ago.

The subconscious processes information rapidly, effortlessly, and automatically. It doesn't have to painstakingly weigh every piece of information like the conscious mind needs to do when making a decision. It's a phenomenon you may have noticed from time to time, and it's one you can learn to harness and use to your benefit.

Perhaps you've noticed your subconscious keeping you safe. You can't put your finger on it, but someone you meet gives you a bad feeling. Or something tells you to pull out of a business deal at the eleventh hour or not to walk down a dark street. The subconscious parts of the brain may make associations with forgotten memories or pick up on things the conscious parts of the brain aren't aware of.

Just as you may have experienced the wisdom of the subconscious when you "went with your gut" in these situations, you may have called upon the power of the subconscious at night, when "sleeping on" something helped you make the right decision.

Perhaps the power of the subconscious surprised you through a particularly meaningful dream. The subconscious loves the wee hours of the morning, when it's free to paint ideas and images across blank canvases, untethered by the shackles and defenses of the logically driven, conscious parts of the brain. Has an important message has ever come to you here? Maybe this dream delivered a universal theme, such as grace or truth, via a symbol of the subconscious. Perhaps this helped you understand some part of your life in a new way.

THE PLAYFUL ONE

The subconscious brain is playful, and it helps you deal with boredom. By daydreaming, it can instantly transport you to Bora Bora, Bali, or Barcelona while you're stuck in a board meeting in Boston. In fact, you can use the subconscious's signature skill of "being somewhere" while simultaneously not being there—as you do when you daydream—to achieve all sorts of goals. In Chapter 4, I'll teach you how to take that existing skill and channel it for different purposes in your life.

The power of what's underneath our everyday frame of mind is potent, is it not? As we will see, it can even be measured by electrodes placed on your scalp—just like a cardiologist may look at your heart by placing them on your chest. When the subconscious is working, slow brain waves are present. They are different than the fast brain waves of the conscious brain that are there when you're working on a spreadsheet.

In many ways, the highly developed, analytical channels of the conscious brain can be seen as both a blessing and a curse for us all. The conscious solves problems animals and small children can't, but with that gift also comes anxiety disorders unique to human beings. It carries some burdens. The conscious has to painstakingly weigh every piece of information to reach conclusions; the subconscious makes instant "gut" decisions. The conscious needs to consume a great deal of energy and willpower to make healthy choices; the subconscious makes it feel like healthy choices happened effortlessly and "all by themselves."

The slow brain waves of the subconscious brain feel really good. That's why so many people like to have a drink to unwind after work. While alcohol is one way to put your mind in an altered state, wouldn't it be nice to learn how to get there without needing to ingest anything to do so? Wouldn't you like to just close your eyes and slow down your brain into a dreamy, trance-like state whenever you'd like? When you learn how to harness the subconscious, this altered, relaxed state can become so much more than just a way to check out. I wonder if you'll be surprised how you can use it to create the happiest and healthiest version of your self.

The subconscious has the power to help you supercharge your future through positively charged suggestions. Which one of your beliefs do you think has set you up for the successes you've already had in your life? The power of beliefs is so incredibly potent, isn't it? Beliefs can set you up to fail or empower you to succeed, so treat them carefully.

People with the most powerful subconscious minds are actually the most open to suggestion, and their brains have a greater abundance of slow brain waves. Beliefs have an even *greater* effect on these people's lives than they do for the average person.

Here's something to consider: the fact that you are reading this book means you are very likely in this category. Highly intelligent, intuitive people who can get immersed in books, plays, films, art, music, or sports tend to have strong subconscious minds with higher-than-average levels of dreamlike brain waves. In the chapters that follow, I'll teach you how to use your uniquely powerful subconscious to your benefit.

GETTING THE LINGO

Before we go any further, it's important for me to explain why I chose the word *subconscious* for the title of this book and the program I created—Subconscious Visualization Technique (SVT). I chose the term subconscious because the tools in this book expand beyond what is sometimes referred to as the unconscious. When I say subconscious, I mean anything that lies below everyday types of thinking.

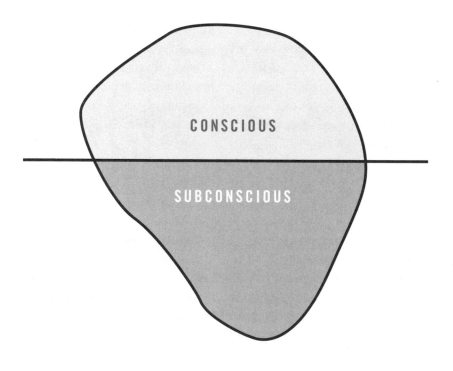

The *Oxford English Dictionary* defines the subconscious as "the part of the mind of which one is not fully aware but which influences one's actions and feelings."[1] Another reference defines it as "that part of the mind which is on the fringe of consciousness and contains material of which it is possible to become aware by redirecting attention."[2] Thus, the subconscious does include what some people may call the unconscious. It includes hidden memories, desires, and drives, and the tools in this book will help you to extract them.

I also prefer the term *subconscious* over *unconscious* because of the subtle differences in their meaning. While the two words can often be used interchangeably, unconscious can sometimes mean sleeping, passed out, or drugged; subconscious does not. It's also important to note that you are not sleeping when you are in a subconscious-dominant state. SVT can be used to treat insomnia; however, it helps you achieve a state that's different from sleeping. You are not unconscious when you use SVT—unless you happen to accidentally fall asleep at some point during the process.

The goal of SVT is to suspend you in the healing potential of subconscious brain waves without falling asleep (when you'd experience *unconscious* brain waves). When you are using SVT, you're in a state that's somewhere in between being asleep and being awake. It's actually much closer to dreaming than it is to sleeping. We can actually use SVT to help you dream while you're awake. And if you're sleep-deprived, a short session of SVT will help you rest and leave you feeling refreshed.

Unconscious can also be interpreted to mean "not conscious," as in unaware or unenlightened. In contrast, SVT—which you'll practice through guided tracks (see page 242)—promotes a conscious and insight-driven way of living. It is a philosophy that empowers you to go out and create the life you were born to live. Before I walk you through the SVT program, I'd like to take you through the scientific proof of the power of the subconscious brain.

Just as I chose to use the term *subconscious* over *unconscious* for the title of this book, I also chose the word *brain* over the word *mind*. While brain and mind are sometimes used interchangeably, your mind is different than your brain. One way many people use these two words implies that changes to the *brain* are clinically measurable, while changes to the *mind* tend to be ones you can perceive without any type of brain imaging to prove it. The word *brain* usually refers to the actual physical structures and, thus, measurable change that is "real." *Mind* implies the nebulous thoughts that many people categorize as less scientific. The way you use the mind can change the

The way you use the mind can change the physical structure of the brain.

physical structure of the brain, and if the physical structure of the brain is damaged, it will affect the way the mind works. The *mind* changes fairly quickly, but to change the activity in the *brain* is a bit more impressive. A few minutes of mindfulness changes the activity of the *mind*; a lifetime of practice thickens structures in the *brain*. By the same token, SVT's effects are so powerful, it's not just the *mind* that changes; it's also the *brain*.

Of course, the mind can also change the brain through your everyday choices. While the brain and mind are both involved in SVT, research using brain scans show that actual physical brain structures get turned on or off by activating the subconscious. When I refer to your subconscious brain, what I'm really talking about is a particular activation of certain brain structures and a deactivation of others—with brain waves moving at a particular speed.

This is no longer just theory; we have the brain scans to prove it. You can see mine on the inside front cover. Many people find that the recent scientific validation of subconscious brain activity increases their buy-in of the treatment, and therefore its effectiveness, even more than personal testimony.

A LITTLE PROOF

Turning on the subconscious brain involves using some specific techniques. It's possible to activate a version of this in animals. For example, a chicken will become mesmerized and immobile if you hold its beak to the ground and slowly draw a straight line away from its beak in chalk,[3] a phenomenon not unlike some of the visual techniques used to activate human beings' subconscious brains. Granted, our brains are more advanced than those of chickens. Yet perhaps the beeps and lights of our iPhones are becoming the chalk that mesmerizes our human brains.

The difference between animals and humans lies in what you can do with the subconscious and the power of suggestion. Scientific research proves over and over the sheer power of suggestion. In fact, subconscious suggestion is the placebo effect that transforms sugar pills into potent treatments.

Research published in 2017 on what's called "open-label placebos" is especially fascinating, since it supports the power of the subconscious and suggestibility. Unlike the traditional placebo study—where the patient doesn't know if he's getting the sugar pill or the drug—open-label placebo studies are those in which patients are actually told, "Yes, you are definitely getting the sugar pill." The doctor delivers this with a positive suggestion, telling the patient that although it is indeed a placebo, it has been shown to produce improvement through healing that originates in the mind. We know that's how placebos work, don't we? A review of five studies showed that open-label placebos—where patients knew they weren't getting any real drug—had a positive effect on IBS, depression, back pain, ADHD, and hay fever.[4] The placebo effect extends even to the pill color because our brains associate certain colors with certain effects, thus making a pill more or less effective.[5]

Another interesting thought to consider: the *side effects* of medication could be partially responsible for subjects reporting symptom improvement in studies. If you were a subject in a traditional placebo, double-blind study—where half the subjects get sugar pills and half get the real antidepressant—the fatigue or nausea you experience could be the clue that you were getting the real drug. This could affect your *belief* that you are taking a powerful drug that is designed to improve your mood. You may in turn be more likely to rate your mood as lifted, thanks to these beliefs. You may wonder if this could create a bias against natural treatments that have fewer side effects where a study compares a natural treatment against a prescription drug. Perhaps a truly unbiased study should give subjects sugar pills that have some sort of side effect.[6]

A few studies have tested using an active placebo with a side effect, but they're rare. If big pharma compared all their drugs in studies head-to-head against active placebos, I wonder how many drugs would actually get approved. It seems drugs' nasty side effects work in their favor through the belief system of your subconscious brain. One thing is certain: the power of your beliefs is potent.

THE "TRICKS" THAT MAKE THE TRADE

Now that you've had a moment to consider what your beliefs can do, you'll learn how to speak directly to your highly suggestible subconscious and how to plant beliefs in your own brain. This "trick" is even more effective when you have activated the slow brain waves of the subconscious through the tools you'll learn in this book.

It's important to know that the subconscious prefers positivity, imagery, and metaphors over negativity and rational reasoning. Rich visuals of healing scenes can be stitched into the parts of the brain that can store traumatic images. This may be partially explained by the fact that hypnosis and guided imagery work thanks to their effect on the right side of the brain,[7] the side that controls your creativity, feelings, and intuition.

The subconscious brain is always looking out for you.

You may realize—as so many of my patients have—that the subconscious brain is always looking out for you. And it helps you tap into the well of strengths and innate capacities that *you already have within you.* Isn't that so nice to know?

I demonstrated the power of the subconscious brain on an episode of *The Dr. Oz Show*. There I was—leading Dr. Oz and his entire studio audience through this subconscious brain–activating practice. I asked them to stare at their hands and told them they'd notice their fingers separate as their subconscious brains became activated. For many people, it feels like this process is happening as if by an outside force. Thus, someone who has never used the practice may think: *Whoa, that's strange. I guess this whole subconscious "thing" actually works . . .*

Then I led Dr. Oz and his audience down a flight of stairs in their minds' eye. On the bottom step, I invited them to find something they needed that day. Would it be a sense of peace? Or would it be a calm type of confidence? Perhaps they'd be reminded of something they forgot. I reminded them that they already had the tools they need to be calm, confident, and courageous.

After all, those inner strengths allowed Dr. Oz to become a top surgeon, didn't they? And what about that single, working mom sitting in the audience? She's a super mom *and* stellar at her job. She already has so much going for her . . . and so do you.

I'll never forget the woman sitting next to us. When Dr. Oz tossed to the commercial break, she whispered to me, "Oh my gosh. That was crazy! I've never experienced anything like that." I could tell by the look on her face that she probably had never activated her subconscious brain before, and she had just had an experience that felt mysterious and magical . . . and quite real. She had turned on a scientific phenomenon inside her brain.

That woman wasn't the only one who had an instant magical experience in mere minutes. When the episode aired, I got a Facebook message from a viewer: "I was watching you on Dr. Oz where you did that subconscious brain thing. What is that?! Meditation has always been hard for me. It makes me more anxious. But what you did on the latest episode you were on made me feel instantly calm. But I can't find the clip online! My brain needs more of that. How can I get more?"

By the time you're done with this book and its practices, I wonder if your experience will be anything like that viewer's. Or will your experience be entirely different?

Maybe you picked up this book feeling like you were seeking someone or something to make you whole or to get you where you need to be. By the time you finish this book, you may end up realizing, like Dorothy in *The Wizard of Oz*, that you had the answers you were seeking all along. As beautiful as the most expensive shoes money can buy may be, your *greatest* power will never be found on your feet. The most powerful tool to change your life is located between your ears.

HACKING THE SUBCONSCIOUS BRAIN

There's a rich visual depiction of the subconscious brain in the movie *Inception*. In this film, Leonardo DiCaprio plays a dream thief who ventures deep into the layers of other people's dreams to steal ideas. He artificially bypasses the defenses of the conscious through the use of an IV drug. Taking the calculated risk of getting stuck there forever, he can hijack others' subconscious brains to steal their contents, a concept known as "extraction."

DiCaprio's character and his team of thieves then pull off a more complicated white-collar crime: subtly planting an idea into a businessman's subconscious brain so that his conscious brain later thinks that he came to this decision himself. This act, known as "inception," would change the course of a corporation's future. The dream thieves discuss the concept: "Once an idea has taken hold in the brain, it's almost impossible to eradicate. An idea that is fully formed, fully understood, that sticks. . . . In a dream state, your conscious defenses are lowered."[8]

Later, they discuss a scientifically accurate concept when it comes to the subconscious brain: positive emotion trumps negative emotion. Remember: the subconscious prefers wonder, possibility, optimism, and positivity, and responds better to such words as *ease* and *comfort*. Modern medicine is a conscious, symptom-based model that focuses on the negative. This can be lifesaving when dealing with acute illness. But when dealing with chronic illness, this approach can begin to train the brain to notice depression, discomfort, and pain.

While some of the concepts in *Inception* are accurate, some are fictional. The dream thieves' need for an IV drug to access their subconscious is one such concept. (No drugs are needed, I promise.) All you need to learn is how to speak to your subconscious with the right type of language and relaxation techniques. However, you won't be able to plant ideas in other people's brains to control them, or take control of Fortune 500 companies, like they did in the film. Sorry about that. However, you *can* plant positive ideas into your own subconscious brain to make them easier to achieve. Whether your goal is healing an elusive condition, boosting the immune system, or creating a career of your dreams, your subconscious can help. Would you like to tap into this profound power? Most people find it's much easier than they even realized.

Once you have activated dreamlike brain waves, you can use positive language, such as "You may be surprised at how easily exercise will begin to feel to you each and every day." That's not sci-fi. It's science. You might notice it tomorrow or sometime next week, but at some point, a thought will bubble up from your subconscious into conscious thought. You'll think: *I'd really like to go for a jog right now.* You may be surprised at how you actually *want* to go for a jog for the first time in years, and you can thank your subconscious brain for the effortless positivity.

DISCOVERING THE PAST

In addition to venturing into the subconscious brains of others, DiCaprio's character also ventures into his own. A rich visual of a vintage elevator with a manual scissor-gate door takes him down as many floors as he'd like to go. Every floor he passes takes him into a deeper memory, with a very dark memory that he keeps locked up on the bottom floor.

Not to worry. For the vast majority of people, the lowest floors simply contain formative, early memories that are quite positive.

You, too, can go on this journey. To do so, you'll just need the right tools to access your subconscious brain.

Step out into a world that's filled with a seemingly infinite number of forgotten memories, abstract thoughts, and ethereal realms to discover. You stumble upon a dusty filing cabinet in some subterranean part of your brain and discover a memory file that you haven't considered in decades. Maybe you had a feeling it was there, or maybe you had completely forgotten about its existence. Perhaps something from that will shed some light on why you're reacting so strongly to something today.

If—like DiCaprio's character—you find a dark memory, I'll show you in Chapter 7 how to delete the file or make it feel less powerful. Perhaps you'd like to move it to another cabinet. Your subconscious has the power to shrink that dark memory and turn mountains into molehills.

Maybe you'll take a pink highlighter and note some of the good things you had forgotten about so that the memory will start to look different from now on. If you wish, your subconscious can rearrange files in a way that will help you to see your life in a more confident and carefree way. Whatever you do with these files, I invite you to venture directly into the subconscious to create deep, profound, and effortless change.

CRAFTING THE FUTURE

In addition to going back into your past, you can use the subconscious to fast-forward and take a glimpse into your future. Rehearse something that hasn't happened yet, and break seemingly impossible tasks into small, achievable microtasks. See how SMART goals—ones that are specific, measurable, achievable, relevant, and time sensitive—unfold step-by-step here. In your waking life, your conscious brain can apply SMART goals to your everyday existence. How much more productive you will be, and how easily will you glide through your days with a sense of calm and confident ease?

Perhaps the subconscious will help you set a world record one day. That's what it did for Olympic gold medal–winning swimmer Alex Baumann. Here's what he had this to say about it:

"In my imagery I concentrate on attaining the splits I have set out to do. About fifteen minutes before the race I always visualize the race in my mind. . . . I think about my own race and nothing else. I try to get those splits in my mind, and after that I am ready to go. My visualization has been refined more and more over the years. That is what really got me the world record and the Olympic medals."[9]

Just as the subconscious brain helped Alex Baumann set a world record, it also helped Dr. Milton Erickson to walk again. He was paralyzed by polio at 17 years old. While recovering and mute, he activated his subconscious brain to slowly teach himself how to talk and walk again.[10] He eventually became a psychiatrist and founded the American Society of Clinical Hypnosis (ASCH), where I completed advanced training in his techniques.

If you're recovering from a traumatic brain injury (TBI), stroke, or car accident, SVT can help you see what you need to do to rewire your brain. Imagery and visualization are powerful tools of the subconscious. In this journey, you may find ordinary time and space begin to disappear—virtual reality using the power of the subconscious brain. It's a visualization in your mind's eye, and it may even feel as if what you're seeing is actually unfolding. The subconscious sees all the manageable steps that need to occur for you to reach your goals, and it can later spoon-feed these in bite-sized pieces to the conscious brain so it doesn't get overwhelmed.

If the subconscious is your iPhone's cloud-based memory with limitless storage potential, the conscious is the small 8 GB memory on the phone itself, with a limited amount of videos, pictures, and apps it can hold at any one time. I wonder how the power of imagery, visualization, and rehearsal will empower you to take control of your life and take action.

POWER PLAY

This subconscious brain-oriented philosophy empowers people to take greater control of their daily lives. In many ways, this helps to shift away from the implied messages of drug companies' ads that are themselves designed to appeal to your subconscious. They're telling you: "Yes . . . you're tired and sick, aren't you? You feel achy and sad, don't you? Yes. That's right . . . you know you do. Our drug will fix you. You know you need it. Take it, and you'll feel as good as this happy, smiling woman." Images are planted in your brain, and they correspond with a belief. You see a woman frowning and aching before taking the pill, and you see her happy after taking it.

How and When to Use SVT

In this book, you'll learn how to use SVT as a self-guided tool. While this is a fantastic skill with a wide variety of benefits for most, some people should not use SVT in this way.

In terms of mental health, self-guided SVT is not a substitute for inpatient or intensive outpatient treatment when major or potentially life-threatening symptoms are present. Some conditions (e.g., anorexia, drug addiction) require a team of professionals wrapping around a person to provide integrative care. SVT may be a tool that becomes part of your treatment plan in an inpatient setting, just like meditation. In acute cases like these, SVT should not be a *substitute* for care—although it can be a great *complement*.

Also, people who have been diagnosed with a major dissociative disorder (e.g., dissociative amnesia, dissociative identity disorder, depersonalization-derealization disorder) shouldn't use SVT as a self-guided tool. I have found SVT to be highly effective for these disorders, but it needs to be delivered in a one-on-one, personalized format. In these acute cases, SVT should only be delivered by a licensed health care professional. Because of its ability to produce visual and auditory hallucinations, don't use SVT if you've been diagnosed with schizophrenia or bipolar I disorder.

In terms of physical health, SVT can complement the healing of elusive conditions, but it doesn't mean you should abandon all your other integrative treatments. Always consult prescribers before making changes to medications or existing treatment plans. Also, SVT can be highly effective at turning off pain. Thus, make sure you rule out major illness first, and *then* use SVT. You don't want to teach the brain to become deaf to an alarm if there's a raging fire present. Pain may be trying to tell you something.

In terms of legal issues, the same rule applies. Get through court proceedings or testimony first, and *then* use SVT. If you are the survivor of abuse or a hit-and-run accident and will need to testify in court, do that first. The subconscious brain is so effective at pressing the delete button and the edit button that your testimony may be deemed inadmissible in court if you have applied your own subconscious's effects to that memory. Once you're through your court date or testimony, then use SVT to choose what *you* would like to delete or edit so that you can set yourself free from any images or memories that are holding you back. It's important to note that the self-guided version of SVT in this book doesn't plant false memories. The only nudging is in the direction of your best interests, positivity, and optimism.

As you are beginning to realize, suggestion is incredibly powerful. While prescription medication can be a piece of the solution for some who truly need it, your everyday choices, your mind-set, your daily diet, your exercise routine, your spiritual practice, the power of hope, and your relationships have an even more profound and lasting role in your health and happiness. On some level, we all instinctually know this to be true. After all, no pill has the ability to force you onto the treadmill, spoon-feed you vegetables, or make you start communicating more openly to your significant other. That's why I'm a strong believer in the behavioral part of cognitive behavioral therapy; our actions are the most important ingredient in the recipe of changing lives. Filling your life with productive, pleasurable, and purposeful events every day is a potent antidepressant, indeed.

The power of combination therapy can help those who already take supplements or medication. If you are taking any prescription medication, supercharge it with the power of your subconscious brain. Perhaps you will find yourself shifting from passive "pill taker" to empowered "go-getter" who makes things happen, and maybe this new place of empowerment will be part of your cure.

TAPPED IN

The SVT program starts with CBT-based tools. In Chapter 3, I'll help you consciously examine the pitfall thought patterns holding you back. In Chapter 4, I'll help you activate your subconscious brain to examine the root of those negative patterns—and break their hold on you.

Then, I'll help you understand the power of something called audio-visual entrainment. This technique, which uses a wearable device, is similar to neurofeedback since it changes brain waves, and it can make very deep subconscious activation possible. The deeper the subconscious activation, the more likely you are to listen to any positivity given to you while in that state. Each chapter after that will help you to target specific areas of concern. For instance, you'll learn how powerful nutrition can be in healing the brain and body. Food truly is medicine, and SVT can help you change how you eat.

Just like anything else you'd practice—piano, skiing, cooking, or basketball—the more you practice SVT, the better you can get. Whether you're a quick study or slow learner, anyone can harness the sheer power of the subconscious brain. It's very rewarding to know that we all have this ability, whether you're a gifted child prodigy or a slow-and-steady pupil.

You may be a neurosurgeon, dog rescue volunteer, or retired housekeeper, but all that really matters is that this program can help you let go of yesterday's woes while ensuring your tomorrow is filled with purpose, power, and productivity. You and I will envision your most incredible future. You'll see yourself manifesting your dreams. Once you're open to suggestion, we'll plant positivity into your subconscious brain. At some point—whether it's tomorrow or next Tuesday—you'll notice your conscious brain implementing the suggestions as if they're second nature. Many people are shocked to find how easily these healthy behaviors become a part of their everyday, conscious life.

No matter your family history or what you've been through, what you choose to do today has the greatest effect on your tomorrow. I wonder what wonderful things you will create and manifest—first in your subconscious and then in your waking, everyday, conscious life. It will be wonderful to see how your actions improve your life and leave this world a better place.

Bonus Material

The Appendix includes bonus scripts of SVT practices for additional areas where you might want the transformative power of your subconscious to help you out, such as overcoming insomnia, deepening spiritual connections, and becoming more successful. Audio tracks of all SVT practices are included with this book; see page 242 for download information.

CHAPTER 2

The Science of the Subconscious Brain

Understanding the groundbreaking science of the subconscious brain—the focus of this chapter—will help you see just how powerful it can be. Comprehending this brain science can supercharge your beliefs, which can help treatments to work even better. When you have a "trippy" experience where you feel like the improvements in your life are happening easily and "like magic," you'll understand the science behind that feeling. And isn't it fascinating to know what's happening inside your brain? That said, this background knowledge is not required for the "brain magic" to work. If you're more a "just give me the goods" person, feel free to skip ahead to the next chapter to start working with the SVT program.

The subconscious brain is a scientifically studied, real part of your brain. It's not just a Vegas sideshow or a fictional thriller. While the tale I'm about to recount may sound like the far-fetched plot of a Hollywood movie, the true-crime story of the Chowchilla kidnapping case demonstrates the scientific power of the subconscious brain—and its ability to access past memories.

In July 1976, 26 school-age students had just enjoyed a field trip to a local pool. On their way home along a country road, their Dairyland Union school bus approached a white van. Then, three armed men jumped out, and the 26 children and their bus driver were forced out of the bus and into two vans. The kidnappers drove the prisoners to a quarry 100 miles away, where a moving van had been buried. The kidnappers forced the children and their driver inside and buried the van with just two air tubes to keep the hostages alive. Then they left to call in a $5 million ransom. Sixteen hours later, the children and their bus driver managed to escape as the kidnappers were sleeping.

When the bus driver was questioned by law enforcement, he wasn't able to remember the license plate of the kidnappers. The FBI called in Dr. William Kroger, a physician who had become well known for his contributions to medical hypnosis. Assisted by Dr. Kroger's hypnosis, the bus driver successfully accessed his subconscious brain and recalled all but one of the characters on the kidnappers' license plate. Justice was served, and the kidnappers all went to prison.[1]

Hopefully, you'll never need to call upon your subconscious to aid in the criminal investigation of a kidnapping. But perhaps you'd like to recall some memories to help you understand who you are in a new way.

Unfortunately, some of the false memory cases of the 1990s, which included false accusations of satanic abuse, used hypnosis (among other techniques) in the patients' sessions. This led to the public's perception that it was the hypnosis itself that created the false memories, rather than the negative and false suggestions the therapists used to influence the patients' subconscious. This phenomenon isn't unique to psychology. It's also found in law—it's why attorneys aren't allowed to lead witnesses during court proceedings. Remember: the mind is, in general, a suggestible entity.

Despite misconceptions about hypnosis and its misuse that make it seem scary, hypnosis won't work without your willingness. The wonder of the subconscious should only be used in your best interests. Use this phenomenon to your benefit with someone who is on your side.

I can't force you to do things you don't want to do, and I can't brainwash you. With your permission, though, this book—or a qualified practitioner—can help painful memories feel more distant and help you become more passionate or productive. If you allow yourself to go with it, the "magic"—if you'd like to use that term—can be a powerful tool indeed. I wonder how this evidence-based program will help you feel better today while helping you create a fantastic tomorrow.

WHAT DO YOU WANT TO DELETE?

The subconscious is remarkably effective at "laying down new tracks" in the brain. If you've seen the movie *Eternal Sunshine of the Spotless Mind,* you may remember the fictional procedure that helped Kate Winslet's character completely forget her ex-boyfriend. She paid a doctor to "delete" the painful memory of her ex to help her through the breakup. Tapping into the power of the subconscious brain may actually be the closest thing to that procedure that exists in modern science.

The subconscious's dreamlike brain waves allow you to "record" a positive memory over a negative memory—at least in the parts of the brain that store images and memories. This can help to change the emotional charge of a memory and get rid of flashbacks and anxiety. Unlike Kate Winslet, you'll still be able to remember who your ex-boyfriend is (sorry about that). You see, the part of your brain that records the facts about your ex remains intact—his name, where he lives, etc. But the part of your brain that records the way you feel about your ex-boyfriend could be slightly altered. If he cheated on you seven times, your subconscious brain can enable you to move on rather than going back to him over and over again.

Would you like to be reminded of how strong and resilient you are? Would you like to take a glimpse into the best-case scenario of your future . . . and see yourself with someone who deserves you? I wonder if you'll be surprised to discover that, through the life-altering magic of the subconscious brain, you may be able to change the way you feel about an ex, a trauma—or any negative experience.

SVT can help you to become more insightful and see your life through a more optimistic lens. Or perhaps you'll come to understand why certain situations or people trigger you in your present life. Many people find great comfort and perspective when they truly understand why their Achilles' heel has been triggered. And with understanding comes the opportunity to heal root causes— once and for all.

Science is in the Scans

The subconscious brain and its power have been used to treat mental illness for centuries. Dr. Franz Mesmer (1734–1815) is credited as being the first physician to demonstrate the brain's ability to change the body via suggestion. The word *mesmerized* comes from his subconscious brain–activating work with his patients. Although his methods, and his hypothesis that this power was magnetic, were discredited (the healing potential had nothing to do with invisible magnetic fluids; it was the way words affected his patients' brains), another physician, Scottish neurosurgeon Dr. James Braid (1795–1860), built on Mesmer's work when he discovered how to put people into trances and came up with the term *hypnosis*. Though the practice had an initially rocky and mysterious start, by the 19th century doctors in India were using hypnosis with patients.[2]

Noted hypnosis researcher Dr. Herbert Spiegel (1914–2009), later a professor of psychiatry at Columbia, used hypnosis to treat traumatized soldiers in North Africa during World War II. He also used hypnosis to treat anxiety disorders and addiction. Despite his techniques being effective and "magical," controversy surrounded their use during Spiegel's early practice.[3] For his part, Dr. Spiegel thanks the "quacks" who, he noted, mostly used hypnosis in the late 1930s. He said, "We are in debt to the quacks for keeping [the practice] alive until the medical community started to investigate and find out what a useful tool hypnotism is."[4]

Spiegel was one of the professionals who helped make hypnosis respectable and reputable, especially for use in medicine. In 1981, Spiegel was quoted as saying, "The prevalent and wrong attitude in the practice of medicine is [to] use a pill or scalpel or a gadget for problem-solving. Modern medicine puts such extreme emphasis on high technology and drugs that it often overlooks the oldest, and at times the most effective, therapeutic instrument that humans possess—the mind. Medicine resorts to it last instead of first."[5] Oh, how true his words remain today.

His son, Dr. David Spiegel, is carrying on his father's work at the Stanford University School of Medicine. He recently published a hypnosis study with brain imaging. There were two fascinating findings. First, hypnosis increased connections between the brain's prefrontal cortex and insula—which may explain how the subconscious brain can control what's going on in the body. Is this why the subconscious can do some things that drugs and the conscious brain can't? Second, the subconscious reduced connections between the brain's dorsolateral prefrontal cortex and the medial prefrontal cortex and posterior cingulate cortex.[6] This is the part people get really excited about, because this makes you blissfully unaware of your actions. When I plant positivity during an SVT practice, you'll later find yourself engaging in this healthy activity without giving it any thought. It will all feel so easy and effortless—as if it just happened. Won't that be nice?

Today, it's these brain-imaging studies that help us to see and understand what is actually happening in the brain when the subconscious is working. Another hypnosis-with-brain-imaging study was conducted by Dr. Amir Raz, the Canada Research Chair in the Cognitive Neuroscience of Attention at both McGill University and SMBD Jewish General Hospital. It led him to conclude that hypnosis can "change focal brain activity in a way no drug we have can do." In this study, subjects were hypnotized and told that the words they would later see would be like "gibberish" and like "characters in a foreign language."

Later, they were given the commonly used research tool called the Stroop test. You may have seen a version of this. It's one of the most famous and widely used tests in modern psychology. The word *green* is printed in red, and the word *yellow* is printed in blue. Because the test activates cognitive conflict in the brain, it's usually difficult to accurately and quickly identify the color. Remarkably, in Dr. Raz's study, the subconscious turned off this naturally occurring phenomenon, and subjects responded as if they were reading words printed in a foreign language. They could name the colors easily and quickly, unlike most subjects given this test.

An fMRI (functional magnetic resonance imaging) brain scan showed what was happening in the subconscious brain: the suggestion given to the subject while in a hypnotic state decreased activity in a part of the brain called the anterior cingulate cortex, a part of the brain affected by the Stroop test.[7] The prefrontal cortex, parietal cortex, thalamus, and insula were also affected. Yes, the subconscious has the unique ability to activate or deactivate all sorts of structures and systems in the brain. Among other talents, it can increase suggestibility, change the sense of time and space, and even create positive hallucinations—or negative ones. Wouldn't it be so nice if vices became invisible to you? As this study demonstrated, that's exactly what the subconscious can do.

> *The subconscious has the unique ability to activate or deactivate all sorts of structures and systems in the brain.*

The subconscious brain has the ability to change the top-down processing that makes sense of sensory data coming in from the bottom up. If you can change top-down processing, then it's more than just a minor reframe in the way you look at something, as you would see in CBT. In fact, you may not be able to see a cigarette or soda can at all. One hypnosis article in *The New York Times* summed up top-down processing quite nicely: "If the top is convinced, the bottom level of data will be overruled."[8]

Change top-down processing, and you may be able to treat the most difficult-to-treat mental illnesses. Instead of being told that words will be like they're written in a foreign language, a smoker could be told cigarettes would become invisible at convenient stores. In all probability, the next time this person was in such a store, he would walk right past the cigarettes and later be surprised to notice how easy this was.

Since these parts of the brain are involved in pain, the subconscious brain can also be used to help with pain relief. In this way, SVT can also help to treat mysterious problems that have some complex and brain-based cause, including the roughly 30 to 60 percent of neurology outpatient referrals who have symptoms that can't be fully explained. For you, I wonder if it could be helpful for exercise to become an enjoyable, easy, and effortless part of your daily routine. Or you may be pleased to find yourself becoming more productive, purpose-driven, confident, and courageous than ever before. This is possible with the help of SVT.

An enlightening 2004 study used fMRI brain scans to demonstrate the sheer power of the subconscious brain.[9] Unlike an MRI, an fMRI can pick up on changes in blood flow and other metabolic changes in the brain. Researchers looked at subjects' brains with fMRIs under three conditions: First, the researchers burned the subjects' hands with a probe heated to 119 degrees. Second, they told the subjects to "imagine" that same pain "as vividly as possible." Third, they used hypnosis to activate the subjects' subconscious brains and then gave them suggestions to "reexperience" the pain to test the power of the subconscious.

The results were amazing: the fMRI showed the brain lit up intensely in the anterior cingulate cortex, insula, prefrontal cortex, and parietal cortex when the subjects had their hands burned . . . or when they used the power of the subconscious brain via hypnosis to reexperience it. However, the researchers saw almost no activation in these parts of the brain when they told the subjects to vividly "imagine" pain, a state that uses conscious channels to re-create and merely "imagine" a sense memory.[10]

Those four brain structures aren't the only parts of the brain the subconscious affects. The subconscious may influence processing at the level of the spinal cord.[11] Research using PET scans (an imaging test using radioactive dyes that are injected, swallowed, or inhaled) found that the subconscious changes the way parts of the brain connect to one another, which affects pain perception.[12]

Another PET scan case study, published in *The Lancet*, showed that this unique pattern of brain activation can be used to temporarily paralyze parts of the body. Similar parts of the brain are involved in patients who have conversion hysteria,[13] a condition where a person's mind is responsible for paralysis. Since the subconscious has the power to paralyze the body, it also means you could use it to help bring body parts back online—something I've done with my own patients. If you're recovering from a stroke, you can use the subconscious to visualize all the microtasks you will undertake to rewire the brain. If you'd like to lose weight, you can imagine yourself on the treadmill every morning—and see that activity taking place in an effortless and easy way.

Would you like to use SVT to simply make sore shoulders feel more relaxed? Hypnotic imagery is even an effective treatment for phantom limb pain, ongoing pain from an arm or leg that has been amputated.[14] The very existence of phantom limb pain in and of itself shows how vital it is to treat the brain as well as the body. Pain coming from a leg that's not there reminds me of one of those Zen riddles about a tree falling in the forest. If no one is there to hear it, does it make a sound? In this case, it does.

Perhaps you're beginning to realize why SVT is powerful in treating pain—and in vividly seeing your future. It's so much more than just "imagining" something. Thanks to the subconscious, the brain actually thinks it's happening. And every time you do something, you create a pathway that lays down tracks of brain cells—and makes any new behavior more likely to continue.

THE MINDBODY CONNECTION

The subconscious brain is so powerful that it can even exert its force on your physical body without the conscious brain realizing it. One study used brain scans and hypnotized subjects while suggesting their hands were being moved by a pulley. Subjects reported they experienced their hands moving as if they were controlled by an external force.[15] Not to worry. The entity that's moving that hand (or helping you to create states of pain-free bliss) isn't something out of *Star Trek* or *The X-Files;* it's your subconscious brain.

If subconscious channels operate below conscious awareness, this also means that positivity planted in the subconscious will probably feel like all that change just "happened effortlessly." Wouldn't it be nice to feel like you just *happened* to effortlessly prefer the fresh fruit over a hot fudge sundae without feeling like you have to consciously push yourself into these—or any other— decisions that are good for you? Wouldn't it be delightful if the woman from work who used to drive you crazy now just reminded you of your patience and grace?

Your subconscious brain can create hallucinations and change the way you perceive time. One Stanford study hypnotized subjects and then suggested they were seeing colors. The researchers could see the parts of the brain that perceive color light up despite the fact the subjects were looking at a black-and-white image.[16] Another study showed how hypnosis visibly affects the parts of the brain involved in your perception of time and space. A few minutes can feel like hours.[17]

Perhaps you're thinking, *Why would I want to create hallucinations or play with time?* Therapeutically, there are lots of reasons. If you can create visualizations and alter consciousness, you can see and hear things the way you wanted them to happen in the past or the way you want them to unfold in the future. The more it feels like a situation is actually unfolding in the present moment, the more you can trick the brain's emotional centers into letting go of traumatic or painful memories from your past. Your old memories will still be there, but their emotional impact will be lessened to a bearable level.

When you're using the subconscious to see every step that needs to unfold to help you create the best future for yourself, that's a beautiful thing. Can you see yourself taking that first step and getting out of this hospital bed? Or see yourself creating the business of your dreams . . . and that move to Chicago you'll manifest next year. You can also use SVT to rehearse a bright future you can look forward to. I wonder what you would like to see—and then how you will manifest these positive visualizations in your waking life.

You may be surprised to learn that the subconscious brain's impact is far-reaching and, thus, can be helpful with conditions that are sometimes characterized as strictly physical or medical in nature. Because the subconscious has access to functions such as digestion, salivation, blood pressure, and your T cells, it can alter things the conscious brain cannot. This has been proven in multiple studies that focused on physical disease, such as one that divided subjects with high blood pressure. The subjects who received hypnosis showed short-term and long-term improvements in blood pressure.[18]

Another study showed the power of hypnosis in treating irritable bowel syndrome (IBS). One group received hypnotherapy, while the other received a standard form of psychotherapy and placebo pills. The patients who received hypnosis showed a dramatic improvement in all IBS symptoms, outperforming those patients receiving standard psychotherapy with placebo pills. In fact, the group who received hypnosis, remarkably, had no relapses after a three-month follow-up.[19]

Your subconscious can also boost your T cells, which fight infection. Ohio State University's Department of Psychiatry, in partnership with the Department of Molecular Virology, Immunology, and Human Genetics, did a study that showed how the subconscious brain boosts the immune system. The subjects were medical and dental students facing their exams—an event so stressful it often affects the immune system. These students learned self-hypnosis and then had their blood tested for T cell count, which is a marker of immune response. T cells went up in subjects who practiced self-hypnosis and went down in those who did not. The more frequently the students activated their subconscious through self-hypnosis, the better the response of their immune systems. This could be seen and validated by the subject's T cell count.[20]

The conclusions of this study are life changing—and not just those of us diagnosed with a condition that directly affects immunity. Why? It shows we can use SVT daily to boost our immune system to fight everything from the common cold to the precancerous cells that are about to spread in our body. Wouldn't you like to experience this for yourself?

RIDING YOUR BRAIN WAVES

The fMRI and PET studies we've been discussing so far show *where* the subconscious works its magic in the brain; EEG studies are better at showing exactly how the subconscious weaves its incredible spells in the brain. An EEG (short for electroencephalogram) measures the brain's electrical signals and brain waves. Generally speaking, you could say it measures how fast or slow your brain is going.

From fastest to slowest, the most common brain waves measured in the human brain are gamma, beta, alpha, theta, and delta. You may have experienced the magic of a fast gamma wave as an "aha" moment. Gamma has been called the *insight* wave.

Beta is the fast brain wave of thoughts, work, and attention. Caffeine and other stimulants increase beta brain waves. Alpha waves are slower and indicate relaxation or light meditation.

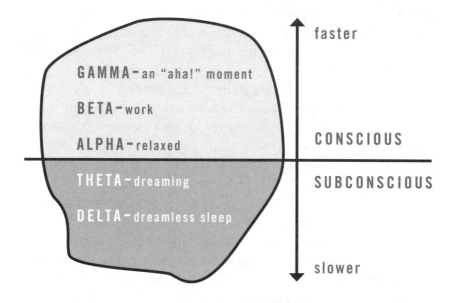

Activate the subconscious, and you can slow your brain waves even more, and you will feel yourself entering a wondrous theta state. Theta is the predominant frequency of children from ages two to five, a time of imaginary friends and easily suspended reality. This also helps explain why subconscious activation helps you access early childhood memories. When you access this frequency, you can use the "spells" of your subconscious brain in ways that serve you.

I liken the subconscious to a five-year-old who sees the world as a magical, wonderful place where dreams come true. She loves wearing her fairy princess costume every day and performing shows for her neighbors. Clinically, her belief in magical worlds and the wonder of possibility makes sense. The subconscious brain increases levels of dreamlike, soothing, slow theta waves.

On the other hand, the conscious brain is akin to a fifteen-year-old who has learned the Tooth Fairy isn't real and pushes back when her parents tell her to be home by 10 P.M. She also tells you she's decided she's not going to college, you're a terrible parent, and she's not trying out for the school play or the volleyball team . . . because she hates *everything* anyway. By this age, the predominant frequency of the brain is alpha—a more conscious, adult, real-world brain wave, which is, of course, far less magical and far more cynical. Alpha lies between the fast beta of working and the deep theta of the subconscious.

The 4/4 time of most music is in the rhythm of theta frequency. In fact, there's even a music genre called trance. Rhythmic drummers tap into this phenomenon. Laser light shows, as well as people swinging light sticks or fire on ropes to the time in 4/4 music, can lull listeners into a captivating state where stressful thoughts seem to disappear. Music can help the brain learn and recover in mysterious ways. As the conscious part of your brain is memorizing cold hard facts, is the subconscious enhancing this effect with Bach or Beethoven? A stroke survivor with aphasia is unable to complete a sentence. Yet that survivor has no problem singing it. Interestingly, both the subconscious brain and music are right-hemisphere dominant. As you'll learn, the subconscious brain weaves most of its spells on the right side of the brain, but SVT also incorporates bilateral stimulation to ensure the left hemisphere is activated as well.

Delta, slower than theta, is the dominant brain wave of infants and deep, dreamless, stage 3 sleep. It can also be seen in the brains of people with head injuries and is more prevalent in the waking state in untreated survivors of childhood abuse.

When you access deep, subconscious information, you use slower brain waves to gain access to them. This helps explain how a name that you consciously stopped trying to remember suddenly pops into your brain. Your subconscious was processing that quest for you, underneath your conscious awareness. Isn't it so reassuring to know that there is an intelligent, instinctual part of you that's always looking out for you?

Research shows that subjects experience a boost in both alpha and theta brain waves—both of which are extremely soothing and relaxing—during and after hypnosis.[21] In many ways, the boost in theta brain waves explains why therapies that access the subconscious brain can work faster or in deeper, more profound ways than traditional talk therapy (like CBT) that works by changing your brain through conscious channels. I'm a fan of CBT. I use it. But in this book, I'll help you supercharge that form of therapy with the power of the subconscious. That's what SVT is all about, merging therapeutic practices—hypnosis, visualization, mindfulness, audio-visual entrainment, and bilateral stimulation—for the most powerful transformation. Your subconscious probably already has its own idea of the spell it would like to weave. The subconscious might have already begun to share this vision with the conscious part of you. Or perhaps it will wait to show it to you during the SVT practice. Either way, your subconscious brain always has one goal in mind: to conspire in the best interests of your happiest, healthiest, and highest self.

Your subconscious brain always has one goal in mind: to conspire in the best interests of your happiest, healthiest, and highest self.

MY SUBCONSCIOUS BRAIN SCANS

You've now learned about published research from a number of different studies. Some studies used electroencephalography (EEG) to measure the speed of your brain waves. Other used fMRIs to measure brain activity and blood flow to the brain.

I asked my friend, best-selling author Daniel Amen, M.D., to help me take a look at the subconscious brain in a way that's never been done. In addition to EEGs, Daniel uses single-photon emission computed tomography (SPECT) scans at his clinics. A SPECT shows activity and blood flow in the brain over the course of minutes. This kind of scan lets us see how SVT is weaving its spells (that is, scientifically valid effects).

A baseline SPECT scan (figure #1, inside front cover) revealed what my brain looked like on a normal day. I spent 20 minutes lying completely still as a space-age machine made its way around my head like a satellite. The next day, Dr. Amen read an SVT script to me (you'll receive the same one later in the book on page 55). Then, we did another SPECT scan (figure #3 on inside front cover) to see if my brain looked any different. I wondered if all this magic was in my head. Well, yes! We could see certain brain structures lighting up like firecrackers.

And what about brain waves? A baseline EEG measured those while my brain was sitting there doing nothing (figure #2)—this time measuring the effects with a different type of technology. This time, I put on a not-so-flattering cap that picked up on electrical signals coming from my brain. Dr. Amen read the same SVT script to me as we repeated the EEG (figure #4). Again, the results were nothing short of remarkable.

Take another look at my before and after brain shots inside the cover of this book. Some of the results were in line with the research you just learned about, but we also made some findings you'll be hearing about for the first time:

The SPECT found:

- Increased blood flow in the basal ganglia, which may help explain why the subconscious has been shown to affect behavior, emotions, and reward systems. Is this why the subconscious brain is so effective at helping people quit bad habits, such as smoking?

- Increased activity in the prefrontal cortex—the most advanced and "human" part of the brain. Is this why the subconscious brain is so effective at treating anxiety, among other concerns?

The EEG found:

- An overall increase in theta brain waves, especially in the frontal lobe. Theta brain waves are responsible for all sorts of revolutionary "brain magic"—from making the "delete" button work better when it comes to trauma to communicating with parts of the body (e.g., the gut–brain axis). Dreamlike theta may help the subconscious access emotional centers of the brain and, thus, work faster than conscious channels. Theta is the signature brain wave of the subconscious, hence the name *Subconscious* Visualization Technique.

- A large boost in beta brain waves in the occipital lobe, which may indicate an immersion in visual worlds painted by the subconscious. Fast beta in the occipital lobe is like virtual reality exposure therapy using the power of your subconscious brain. Your eyes may be closed, but your subconscious brain is *seeing* that cat you used to fear. Or it's seeing you build the business of your dreams, walking into that boardroom with cool, collected confidence—step-by-step. Paired with the evaporation of your sense of time, SVT allows you to rehearse the entire sequence in just a few minutes. And if the brain thinks it's seeing it, then it's "real" to the brain. Beta in the occipital lobes is true visualization, hence the name Subconscious *Visualization* Technique.

UNDERSTANDING THETA

The multitalented theta brain wave is restorative in mind and body. Theta helps both the brain to release feel-good neurotransmitters and you to focus. That's because these brain waves have the power to shut down other frequencies, keeping your brain on task. Theta is like a stern headmistress who keeps rowdy students in line. Generally speaking, the subconscious brain bathes the brain in theta. But some areas of the brain may actually see boosts in fast beta while others are being soothed by theta. And it's possible to see a gamma brain wave, the signature of the "aha" moment, pop up between theta waves.

If you don't have enough slower brain waves, like alpha and theta, and instead have more fast beta brain waves, you're likely to have excess levels of the stress hormone cortisol. Having an abundance of the fast brain waves makes you more likely to develop PTSD.[22] Pain is also associated with higher levels of beta brain waves,[23] so the ability of hypnosis to relieve pain is partially thanks to an increase in theta. EEG studies have even shown how the ability of animals to change their brain waves resulted in a corresponding spike in other feel-good neurotransmitters, such as dopamine.[24]

Theta brain waves help you recall the past, and when they are harnessed properly, it becomes easier and more effective to rescript the past and your future. The theta brain wave also allows both the "delete" and the "record" buttons in your brain to work better. Here's why: Theta brain waves are the footprint of the subconscious and can travel throughout the brain, unlike conscious brain waves (e.g., beta), which tend to stay in one area. Theta brain waves are also the dominant brain wave in the brain's amygdala and hippocampus, which are the brain's centers of emotion and memory. I have found that when it comes to PTSD, getting over your ex, taping over a memory, or just becoming less anxious, tapping into this part of the brain and theta brain waves is faster and more effective than using conscious brain waves to reach the same goals.[25]

This research helps us understand how practicing SVT can help you become happier or healthier via your subconscious brain. It may also help you understand how you may have developed a problem in the first place. I wonder if the improvement, and how quickly it will begin to unfold, will surprise you.

Not surprisingly, patients diagnosed with PTSD who learned how to generate more theta brain waves reported fewer symptoms.[26] Research also shows that alcoholics who learn to generate more theta brain waves were much more likely to stay sober. SVT will teach you to produce more theta brain waves. And even if trauma and addiction aren't concerns for you, SVT can help all people to stress less and feel increasingly calm in body and mind. In one study, alcoholics were divided into two groups. Ten got standard care, including a 12-step program and traditional psychotherapy. Ten got a type of therapy that helped them increase theta brain waves. That second group was less likely to relapse 13 months later and experienced a sharp reduction in depression.[27]

Another study divided inpatient substance users into two groups; 77 percent of the group that learned to generate theta brain waves was abstinent a year later, compared to 44 percent of the group that did not.[28] These clear statistics show you how powerful the subconscious brain can be—even in cases of addiction with high rates of relapse.

And if you want to boost your creativity, theta can certainly help you. When you fall asleep, your brain passes through dream-like theta as it transitions from faster beta and alpha brain waves on its way down into delta, which is associated with deep, dreamless sleep. That's what may have helped Thomas Edison invent the light bulb. It's been said that when he couldn't crack a problem, he would nap holding ball bearings in his hand. When he started to fall asleep, he would drop the bearings and wake himself up. He'd then find himself able to resolve whatever problem his conscious brain had been having trouble solving. Thomas Edison knew that his supremely creative mind could literally "invent the light bulb"; it was in the theta brain waves of his subconscious. Wouldn't it be nice if SVT helped you create more of those wonderfully relaxed theta brain waves that helped Thomas Edison light up our world, so you can light up yours?

If you want to boost your creativity, theta can certainly help you.

Blisstul Rest

SVT can also help boost theta while you're awake. Why is this helpful? Clinically, the theta brain wave, which is associated with dreaming and REM sleep, is healthy and restorative for your brain.

One 2017 study found that people who spent more time in REM sleep had lower fear-related brain activity the following day.[29] REM has been shown to affect the levels of neurotransmitters (chemical messengers) in your brain. The authors of another recent study found that the part of the brain that secretes stress hormones actually takes a break during REM sleep, concluding, "The more REM, the weaker the fear-related effect." The researcher went on to explain, "It affects the degree to which the amygdala—the fear center of the brain—is sensitive to stimuli."[30]

REM clearly exerts powerful stress-relieving effects on the brain. Like REM sleep, SVT is also theta brain wave dominant. Both states are marked by noticeable eye flutter that may correspond with activity in the occipital lobe, the fear center, and both hemispheres of the brain. In other words, you are simultaneously *seeing* it, *feeling* it, and *making sense* of it. If dreaming helps the brain to discharge traumatic memories, then SVT can be thought of as a type of dreaming that occurs when you're awake. While you have little or no control over the content of your dreams while sleeping, SVT can be thought of as a type of controlled dreaming.

READY TO TRY SVT?

Part of you—maybe your subconscious—now believes in the science of what SVT can do for you. You know there was a reason you picked up this book, don't you? I will show you how to activate your subconscious brain . . . and how to tap into the true magic of this evidence-based practice for sustainable success. What would you like to heal, dream, or manifest now that you understand the power of your sensational subconscious brain?

CHAPTER 3

A Conscious Start to Subconscious Healing: SVT Step 1

At this point, you're probably excited to start using the power of your own subconscious brain. Which healing or aspirational aspect appeals to you most? Would you like your subconscious brain to help your body feel comfortable? Your subconscious can neutralize the conscious brain's tendency to look for the evidence of pain—and the worst-case scenario of what that pain could mean.

Would you like your subconscious brain to help you feel more confident, creative, and calm in business? Your subconscious can neutralize the conscious brain's obsession with what negative things other people may be saying about you. The subconscious wonders what your colleagues like about your presentation. I'll teach you to plant a suggestion: "At some point in your presentation, you'll notice a feeling of cool, calm, confidence coming over you. I wonder when that will be . . ." Perhaps sooner than you expect, you'll enjoy how naturally and easily it then happens for you.

You're probably starting to understand how the conscious brain holds you and your subconscious back, like a stern parent who stifles a creative child.

> **The subconscious brain:** "Mom, I want to audition for the school play!"

> **The conscious brain:** "No! Sit in your room and finish your math drills. Do you know how hard it is to get into Ivy League colleges these days?!"

Of course, what's important is that SVT integrates both the subconscious *and* the conscious brain. SVT will help you say: "Audition for the school play and finish your math homework. I wonder what extraordinary career using *both* sides of your brain will lead you to one day!"

Perhaps right now, the only time your subconscious brain gets to play is during your dreams. Wouldn't it be great to be able to tap into this healing potential during your waking hours? In steps 6 and 7 of SVT (Chapter 5), I'll teach you how to connect what you discover through your subconscious brain with everyday, waking *behaviors*. The subconscious will weave the dreams, and then the conscious will help you manifest them. SVT will help you see the career of your dream unfold step-by-step. Then, rise and grind to make what you saw your new reality.

But first, the conscious

Before beginning this journey into the subconscious, it's important to take another look at the conscious part of the brain. Why? Research shows that subconscious brain–based practices can double the effectiveness of CBT.[1] Thus, it's not a matter of using the subconscious or the conscious brain. Rather, for optimal results we should utilize a synergistic approach—combining the best of old-school, rational CBT with the innovative, subconscious-based practices you'll use with SVT.

Step 1 of SVT starts with a cognitive, conscious brain–based exercise—and you'll complete this step in this chapter. We'll also come back to it in the condition-specific chapters in the second part of this book. As you complete step 1, let me tell you two interesting things I believe will be happening in your brain as I would view it in brain scans. The first has to do with which *side* of your brain lights up, and the second has to do with the *speed* of your brain waves. Let's unpack these one at a time.

Early on, there was an idea that the subconscious brain worked by lighting up the right side of the brain. In the 1970s, two EEG studies by the same researcher who had this theory couldn't find evidence to support it, but then three other researchers in the 1980s and 1990s *did* find evidence that the subconscious brain indeed turns off the left side of the brain and activates the right side of the brain.[2]

When you employ your conscious brain to analyze your life, you are using the rational *left side* of your brain. So before we start harnessing the intuitive wisdom of the right side of your brain in step 2, let's not forget what the rational left side of your brain has to say here in step 1. Step 1 and the guided journal entry at the end of this chapter likewise use conscious brain–based reasoning to determine which of seven pitfall thought patterns hold you back. Then, the next steps of SVT will help you break free from those pitfall thought patterns by using the subconscious brain, which you'll practice in Chapter 7.

In the next chapter, you'll learn how to activate the subconscious brain—this is step 2 of SVT. Research shows that subconscious activation lights up the *right side* of your brain. And just as it helps you integrate these two sides of your brain, it helps balance who you are.

Now let's talk about the *speed* of your brain waves. In Chapter 2, you learned how the subconscious slows most of your brain down into theta brain waves, the same ones an EEG would record while you're dreaming. The conscious brain uses faster beta brain waves, shown on an EEG when you're alert or working on a problem. You also learned that a concentration of beta brain waves indicates anxiety, so we don't want your brain to get stuck in these fast brain waves. SVT is remarkably effective because it teaches your brain to speed up *and* slow down. It's like interval training for your brain. You don't get "stuck" in either type of brain wave, either. You can, for example, use theta to brainstorm an idea and then use beta to work on the spreadsheet that will help support the financial structure of that idea.

THE SEVEN PITFALL THOUGHT PATTERNS

Here in step 1 of SVT, you're using the beta brain waves of the conscious brain. Now it's time to learn about the seven pitfall thought patterns. Many of these pitfall thought patterns correspond with excess beta brain waves or an inability to move easily from one brain wave to another. These patterns are associated with depression, anxiety, fear, and living below your potential. I invite you to begin by considering which ones are holding *you* back in your everyday life.

Most people tend to struggle with a few of these seven pitfall thought patterns in particular. People with anxious brains will often identify with paralysis by analysis (also known as rumination) and pessimism (also known as worst-case-scenario or catastrophic thinking). If you struggle with confidence or depression, perhaps personalization is holding you back. Introverts tend to wrestle with psychic thinking since they often find it difficult to verbalize feelings—and, in doing so, they expect others to read their minds.

Here are the seven pitfall thought patterns and an example of how they may sound in a person's mind. As you read this list, notice if any of them sound familiar to you.

1. **Paralysis by analysis:** This type of thinking involves stewing and ruminating in anxious thoughts, preventing productive action from occurring. For example: "I wonder why Alex got that account and not me. Does my boss like him better than me? I wonder if it's because of that mistake I made last

month on that account. My boss said she wasn't mad, but maybe she was and just didn't want to tell me. She did give me a funny look this morning. I should be focusing on that other project right now, but I just can't stop thinking about this . . ."

2. **Permanence:** This thought pattern falsely assumes that just because something is a problem now, it will always be a problem. Mood-congruent recall is a phenomenon in the brain that lights up similarly charged memories. If this charge is negative, it will create the illusion that you've always been sad or anxious and, therefore, will always be sad or anxious in the future. For example: "I just can't move on from losing my cat Mittens. I know it's been a year, but I still cry every time I think of her. It just feels like I'm never going to get over this. I'm never going to be a happy person ever again."

3. **Personalization.** This mind-set is when you tend to blame yourself if things don't go your way, even when that result has absolutely nothing to do with you. Dirty looks from a coworker are sometimes just the result of him having a really bad day—not because he dislikes you. Other times, you put all the blame on yourself when there are multiple people, as well as circumstances, involved in the unfavorable outcome. While there may be things you'd like to have done differently, it does take two to tango. Disagreements, divorces, and disasters are rarely *entirely* one person's fault. For example: "I sent out three resumes and didn't get any calls. What's wrong with me?"

4. **Pervasiveness:** This perspective is the difference between seeing a negative event as something that is global versus something specific. If pervasiveness takes over, your thinking becomes global—and something bad in one area of your life has now spread

to all areas of your life. For example: "I can't believe I weighed that much at the doctor's appointment today. That just put me in a really bad mood. I feel like giving up on everything now. I was going to work on the new business I was planning to start, but I don't feel like it anymore. And as for tonight's plans, I'm going to text my friends and cancel that dinner. I'm just going to stay home and order a pizza."

5. **Pessimism:** This type of thinking considers the worst-case, catastrophic scenario. It dwells in the possible, not the probable. For example: "If my daughter doesn't have a child soon, I read she's going to be considered a high-risk pregnancy. I'm worried that she's going to die during childbirth if she waits until she's thirty. If she waits any longer, she'll have to take hormones. I've read that can give women cancer. My daughter is going to die young! Oh, gosh . . . this is so terrible."

6. **Polarization:** This mind-set has a binary, black-or-white pattern. The words *always* or *never* are frequently found in your thoughts and your words. For example: "If I fall off my healthy eating regimen at any point during the day, my *entire* day is *totally* ruined!"

7. **Psychic thinking:** This type of thinking either assumes that the other person is psychic—so he or she has to read *your* mind without you verbalizing what you need—or vice versa. When you assume you are psychic, even though the other person hasn't verbalized something, you think you know what he or she is thinking. And, of course, you assume the worst. For example: "Why did my husband just do that? Doesn't he know I had a hard day? It would have been nice for him to cook dinner tonight. Fine! I'll just do it myself . . . and when he asks me what's wrong, I'll just say, 'Nothing!'"

Identify your top three pitfalls and circle them:

1. Paralysis by analysis

2. Permanence

3. Personalization

4. Pervasiveness

5. Pessimism

6. Polarization

7. Psychic thinking

Now write an example of how each one of these pitfall thought patterns frequently sounds to you.

My Top 3 Pitfall Thought Patterns:

1. Type of pitfall thought pattern: _____

   _____

   which, to me, is a thought that sounds something like:

   _____

2. Type of pitfall thought pattern: _____

   _____

   which, to me, is a thought that sounds something like:

   _____

3. Type of pitfall thought pattern: _____

   _____

   which, to me, is a thought that sounds something like:

   _____

CHANGING YOUR MANTRA

Does your brain deliver to you a negative, one-sentence mantra? For many, this negative mantra may be a version of their most distressing and dominant pitfall thought pattern. In other people, this negative mantra may reflect the underlying essence of all their top three pitfalls. A negative mantra may be omnipresent in your day-to-day life, or it may come and go. You may notice that your negative mantra tends to get louder when you are struggling the most.

Whether you are consciously aware of it or not, your pitfall thought patterns have contributed to a negative mantra that is charged with emotion. This negative mantra affects the way you are in the world, how you see it, and how you behave in it. In the brain, thoughts, feelings, and actions all go hand in hand. You may be currently walking around with a mantra that says: "I'm unlovable." "I'm not good enough." "Something's wrong with me." These are common negative mantras. Negative mantras can fuel negative beliefs, becoming "truth" to *both* your conscious and subconscious brain. What is the primary negative mantra you'd like to be free of?

Whether you are consciously aware of it or not, your pitfall thought patterns have contributed to a negative mantra that is charged with emotion.

Negative mantra that's no longer serving me: _____

_____

_____

Throughout this program, it will be inspiring to see how you change any negative mantra into a positive one. I wonder what confident, carefree, purpose-driven, and positive mantra you'd like to create in the old one's stead. Perhaps you'll see your mantra change in these ways:

- "I'm not good enough" is transformed into "I'm a confident, caring, and courageous person."

- "What's wrong with me?" becomes "I'm so proud of everything I've already done in my past, and I can't wait to go create more 'right' in my bright future."

- "I'm unlovable" turns into "I am truly worthy of love."

SVT will help you to perform the evidence-based alchemy necessary to create this transformation. Consider all this for a moment, and then write your new positive mantra in the space below. As you work your way through the SVT program, it will be astonishing to see how your subconscious makes this positive mantra your reality.

The new, positive mantra that I will manifest is: _____

_____

_____

As we work through specific problems and conditions in upcoming chapters, we'll return to step 1 to determine which pitfall thought patterns are playing a role in fear, anxiety, mood, insomnia, pain, health, spirituality, and success. We'll explore the science so your conscious brain is on board, then, with awareness and SVT, we'll let your subconscious do the rest of the work. Aren't you curious to see how easily change for the better takes hold? Here we go: a subconscious-led journey to your happiest, healthiest, and highest self.

CHAPTER 4

Activating the Subconscious Brain: SVT Step 2

Now the fun part begins. You've already used your conscious brain to examine the pitfall thought patterns and negative mantras holding you back—step 1 of SVT. Let's turn your attention to the heart of SVT, steps 2 through 7. These steps tap into the power of your subconscious brain.

In the second part of this book, we'll repeat these steps of SVT in different ways to specifically target goals you may have—from weight loss to boosting mood to taking your business to the next level. While step 1 was done as a stand-alone journal exercise, steps 2 through 7 of SVT are done as a single practice with no starts and stops.

BRAIN MECHANICS

While step 1 of SVT used the conscious brain in an analytical way, steps 2 through 7 keep you immersed in the subconscious.

This means a few things are going on in your brain. You'll feel the shift as the brain begin to slow down from beta brain waves to the dreamlike theta brain waves and you shift from using the left side of your brain to using its right side. You're turning on and off certain brain structures: the prefrontal cortex, the basal ganglia, the occipital lobe, and the anterior cingulate cortex, just to name a few. Collectively, these changes show you are now using your *subconscious* brain. The subconscious is even increasing the connection between your prefrontal cortex and the insula, tapping into the brain's control of what's going on in your body. This may explain why activating the subconscious can help heal IBS and migraines. At the same time, the subconscious decreases the connection to the anterior cingulate—your worry center. Aren't you curious to find out how your subconscious will help you?

STEP 2: ACTIVATING THE SUBCONSCIOUS WITH THE 3/12/7 METHOD

First, let's unpack step 2 so you can experience activating the subconscious. You'll use The 3/12/7 Method script (see page 55) to slow down your brain, shift it from left- to right-hemisphere dominance, and turn on and off different parts of the brain.[1] By deactivating the defenses of the conscious, you'll start to notice how easy it is to access the deepest, most joyous wells of healing and potential to manifest an incredible future in the steps of SVT that follow. SVT is a learned skill; the more you use it, the more deeply you will activate your subconscious. Not only that, but you'll also engage your subconscious brain more quickly, and the positive transformation will stick.

I recommend that you use SVT at least a few times a week. Multiple studies have demonstrated that benefits amplify as subjects use subconscious-activating practices more. After you practice SVT once or twice, you'll probably feel something happening in your brain. After you practice it eight times, you'll probably notice changes in your body or subtle changes in the way you talk to yourself. After you've been practicing it for a year, your life may look and feel significantly different than it does today. If you are experiencing the pain of daily migraines or the disaster of a messy divorce, then you can even use SVT as a daily tool. Think of SVT as you would a meditation practice: the more you use it, the greater the benefit.

Need a Quick Recharge?

Since SVT boosts dreamlike theta brain waves—the same brain waves that occur during REM sleep—you can actually use a short practice of SVT as a "nap" on days when you didn't sleep well the previous night. While nothing beats a solid eight hours, REM and dreams only happen in your last few hours of sleep.[2] Dreaming and SVT isn't just spinning leftover wool into throwaway pieces of yarn. Not getting enough REM sleep time has recently been associated with both dementia and depression.[3] Since SVT harnesses the same brain waves as dreams, it may even be a way to promote better brain health.

As you'll see in the written scripts and the audio recordings available for download (see page 242), step 2 begins by using a type of mindfulness meditation to center your brain. This first part of The 3/12/7 Method will take most brains from beta down into slow alpha brain waves. Being alert is associated with beta brain waves; meditation is associated with alpha brain waves.

Then, in steps 3 through 7, I add many subconscious-based techniques to expand The 3/12/7 Method. These include hypnosis, guided imagery, visualization, and cognitive-behavioral techniques. This combination slows down the brain from alpha to dreamlike theta. This is why many people say that hypnosis feels "deeper" than meditation.

Most people will find this book's special audio tracks to be the easiest way to begin activating the subconscious brain. I strongly encourage you to start with them. As you become more skilled at activating your subconscious brain, you may wish to review the written script. The more you use SVT, the more you will be able to memorize the script and recite it silently to yourself to activate your subconscious brain without the audio tracks, if you'd like.

You'll read the full version of The 3/12/7 Method in just a minute, but the more you use it, the more you'll be able to short-hand the script. Just like an elite athlete with muscle memory, you will begin to capture the essence of what it feels like to enter into this state. You will probably become so skilled at activating the subconscious brain that you will enter into this state more quickly every time you do so. Many people find they can eventually do so in a single second or two. However, allow yourself enough time for a full SVT practice of steps 2 through 7. I suggest setting aside 20 to 30 minutes and using it at the end of your day so you don't try to rush through it.

I often create personalized SVT recordings for people to enhance their healing or business potential. In doing so, I ask them to tell me if they prefer the image of an elevator or stairs. Do you like beaches or meadows?

If someone hates confined spaces but loves the beach, I won't use a small elevator in the script and will instead use imagery such as a beach or a series of descending rooms as a replacement. Then, I assess this person's most important goals and put those into the recording. These personalized tracks help to optimize subconscious activation and healing.

I provide several tracks as part of The 3/12/7 Method. The default audio track (and script on the following pages) uses stairs, but each track and script in Chapters 7 through the Appendix use other images. Try them all and see which you prefer. As you become proficient at using SVT, you can begin to replace my words or images with ones that are most pleasant or calming to you. Or you may want to recite your own script in your mind.

Feel free to read the script now, but when you're ready to practice activating your subconscious, close your eyes and listen to the audio track. Down the road, if you choose to memorize the script to make it your own, take your time to visualize each part of the journey with your eyes closed. The goal of going only through step 2 right now is to let you experience the relaxing, creative wonder of activating the subconscious.

The script below is a blueprint that you can customize with any imagery that works best for you, using your creative, subconscious brain. After you go through the experience of activating your subconscious, I'll also show you how to deactivate it in case you need to return to daily activities.

Note: At some point during The 3/12/7 Method, the images, memories, and visions are likely to become vivid. Many people feel more at ease by simply reminding themselves that they are the observer watching from a comfortable distance—as if you're in a theater watching a scene on a stage. Later, you'll also learn how to change that scene so that you have a greater sense of control over what you see and experience.

THE 3/12/7 METHOD

In a comfortable seated or lying posture, listen to audio track "The 3/12/7 Method" to experience the simple activation of your subconscious brain (see page 242 for download instructions and codes).

I'd like you to begin with a simple invitation to your own subconscious, asking it to help you in this journey of deep relaxation and healing. I invite you to begin this practice by allowing the eyes to close as you settle in here . . . as the body finds the most comfortable position to rest.

As you start to relax your mind and body, notice how you already know the best way for you to relax, how you like to position the body, whether you're sitting or reclined if that's more comfortable. How do you like to position the hands and the legs?

As soon as you are ready to begin relaxing more fully, you may notice the body making any last adjustments it needs to enhance this journey to healing, happiness, and your highest self.

In just a moment, but not quite yet, I'll lead you through a series of specific steps that will help you to activate the subconscious brain in an even more profound way.

Maybe you've already noticed yourself settling down into a more restful state . . . or perhaps you'll begin to notice it in just a few moments. As your conscious hands over control of the body to the subconscious in this journey, you may even notice a slight twitch in the body, the mouth watering, or the body becoming bendy—just as you may experience when you're sleeping, dreaming, or napping. These are all simply indications that this surprising brain magic you've just learned about is working. At some point in this practice, you may even notice a flutter in the eyes as though you're dreaming—yet another indication that the subconscious brain is working.

*Now I invite you to start your journey with mindfulness, which is simply an awareness of the present moment. Start by using your sense of hearing. Pay attention to three **sounds** you can hear right here and right now. It could be interesting to move from the loudest sound you're hearing to the faintest one you're perceiving . . . right here and right now. I wonder what the loudest sound is . . . right here and right now. Now, what is a sound that's neither loud nor soft? And now . . . a soft sound. Can you hear your heart beating or your breath breathing? That's right. Perfect.*

*Now I invite you to pivot your attention to your sense of sight. Isn't it so interesting that even with the eyes closed, you can still see color on the back of the eyelids? Just notice **two colors**—the first being a color on the back of the eyelids straight out in front of you. Then, on your next inhale, see a color up near the crown of the head as you roll the eyes up, up, up. Perfect.*

*On the next exhale, allow the eyes to float down, down, down . . . and then just allowing the eyes to relax . . . allowing any lingering tightness to float away. Yes, that's right. And now I invite you to really feel **one breath**. Can you feel where the next breath enters your nostrils? Can you feel the temperature of the air as you breathe in? Can you feel the breath? Isn't it so nice to know that the breath is always there—like the subconscious brain—always taking care of us? Always rocking us . . . like a mother rocking her baby. That's right. Perfect.*

As you tune in to your senses rooted in this present moment, you will probably find that the judgment, scrutiny, and defenses of the conscious begin to float away. Does this make your experience even more relaxing? As we continue here, I invite you to simply allow this experience to unfold, and as it unfolds, know that the subconscious has always been here looking out for you—yes, your subconscious has your back and always has. You know that now, don't you?

Throughout this process, it's not even necessary to listen carefully to the words you may be reading or hearing now . . . because the subconscious is perceiving and responding to everything that is read or said—without any deliberate effort on your part. After all, that's how the subconscious brain works. It may feel like a part of you is drifting off to a far-off place in your awareness as some other part of you is hearing every word I say. Isn't that so nice to know?

As you're now already activating your subconscious brain, you may be surprised at the rediscovery of a kind of optimism. Perhaps a sense of childlike wonder comes to you at some point in this process. I don't know if you're feeling it already or if you'll feel it a bit later.

Whenever you discover a piece of that, you'll realize that the subconscious is always looking out for you—it sees your greatest potential today and sees what possibilities you can look forward to tomorrow. Some part of you already knows this, doesn't it? Isn't it so nice to be reminded of this?

Throughout this healing journey, you will probably find that images and memories are more vivid and lifelike when viewing them through the lens of the subconscious. You can take comfort in the fact that, here in this safe space, you are the observer of everything that unfolds. In the real world or in your dreams, you have less control. But here, you are in control of what you see and how you see it.

Many people find comfort in the fact that they are merely viewing the images, memories, and visions they experience. Since you're the observer, it may feel like you're an editor . . . you're using a computer to view and edit a film on a screen.

This movie can become 3D, all-encompassing, and lifelike if you'd like, but the subconscious—in its never-ending mission to look out for your best interests at all times—also knows if it needs to bring some part of you back . . . distancing you from anything you see, hear, and experience here. Isn't it so nice to know that, as the observer of this healing process, you always have the power to ground yourself?

Also, you have the power to bring yourself out of this at any time. . . . Isn't that so empowering? I invite you to send a message to the subconscious that today, you're only going to see, hear, and experience what you're ready to see, hear, and experience. . . . Call upon the subconscious right now, and softly ask it to help you in the way you most need today.

Isn't it so nice to know your subconscious is conspiring in your favor and always knows what you need to heal and grow? Remember, your subconscious is responsible for your gut feelings and intuition . . . so it has a deep sense of what's right for you.

In just a moment, but not quite yet, you'll use the power of your mind's eye to see and feel yourself going down an elevator. I wonder what wonderful healing is in store for you today. Now I invite you to use the full creative potential of the subconscious to use the mind's eye in the next step in this journey.

In just a moment, but not quite yet, you'll use the power of your mind's eye to see and feel yourself going down an elevator with **12 floors.** *You'll feel so delightfully dreamy and deep by the time you reach the first floor. See yourself at the top of this elevator. That's right. Is it one of those old-school elevators with a scissor gate or a modern one? I wonder if it is silver or gold or white? You already have a sense coming to you now that this journey will be a safe and healing one.*

Visualize yourself stepping into that elevator and pressing the number one with your finger. Perfect. In just a moment, you'll begin to feel your body descend. And when that happens, you'll notice that your mind begins to feel more and more relaxed.

12. *Begin to feel a deep sense of restorative healing washing over you. That's right.*

11. *As you feel the elevator descend, you'll become twice as relaxed as the floor before.*

10. *Simply allow the body to take all the time it needs. Many people notice the breath becoming slower and more relaxed here. I wonder if you may notice your breath moving down into your belly as it does when the subconscious begins to take over. That's an indication that you're more relaxed. As the breath slows, the mind calms.*

9. *I wonder if you can actually feel a sense of the body moving down. And as you do, you're becoming more calm and comfortable.*

8. *Perhaps noticing now how this relaxation may help you to let go of any tightness in your body. And as that happens, your mind easily lets go of any remnants of conscious thought or worry. That's right. Good.*

7. *Even deeper now. It's almost as if, with every floor you descend, you become two or even three times more relaxed and comfortable than you were on the floor before. And when that happens, I wonder if you'll just notice how nice it all feels.*

6. *Halfway down now. That's right. Letting go a bit more now. Isn't that such a nice feeling? Lean into it too now. Do you feel the body becoming a little heavier or a bit limp as the subconscious brain allows your body to feel so free? You deserve this rest. You do so much in your everyday life, don't you?*

5. *Almost there now, and you may notice that the mind embodies the same easy "rag doll" quality as you may feel now in the body. Your mind no longer has to do anything. I wonder if you have already begun to feel like there's something that you were meant to let go of today. Either way, it can be so incredible just to have this time to rest, relax, and recharge.*

4. *Feeling yourself move to the next floor down, you may notice a wonderful dreamlike state come to you—now or at some point in this journey. And you have a sense that everything you're going to experience here is going to be so healing. Isn't that nice to know?*

3. *Almost there now. That's right. You're doing so wonderfully already . . . and you've only just begun.*

2. *Next-to-last floor. Perfect. Feeling twice or maybe even three times as calm, dreamy, or relaxed on this step as you were on the floor before.*

1. *Notice now . . . where in the brain or body do you feel the most relaxed? If you'd like, allow that relaxation to spread over the rest of you, especially to the place you need it most. Just take all the time you'd like here to enjoy this type of experience you're feeling now. That's right. Very good.*

*Now that you've felt the **body** make its way down the elevator, you've probably noticed the **brain** begin to slow itself down into a state of healing relaxation.*

*In just a moment, you'll feel the **body** start to float upward as your **consciousness** begins to expand—as I count up from one to seven. As these two things happen—**body floating** and **consciousness expanding**—you may notice an even deeper sense of peace and relaxation.*

As the body floats, many people also notice it feels warm—as though you're taking a warm bath or floating in the ocean on a summer day. And as you practice this more, you may even find that you lose a sense of time and space. You may even find that if you'd like you can create a sense of "leaving" the physical body for this healing time you've given yourself. If it feels comfortable, you may wish to see your consciousness actually leaving the physical body as a momentary kind of "out-of-body" experience. If you'd like, you can see your consciousness moving upward toward the sky and leaving the physical body.

Counting now:

1. Body float.

2. Consciousness moving upward and expanding so that it's now larger than the body.

3. Body becoming lighter and warmer.

4. Consciousness moving upward and expanding even more so that it fills the room.

5. Body becoming almost weightless now.

6. Consciousness so elevated and expanded that it's joining with the universe.

7. So deep and so relaxed. Perfect.

DEACTIVATE THE SUBCONSCIOUS

Now that you've learned how to activate your subconscious brain, it's important to learn how to deactivate it. If you are using SVT in the middle of the day, you'll need to speed your brain back up to the faster beta and alpha waves associated with daily life. If you "stay down" in the subconscious, your brain will continue to oscillate in slow theta brain waves.

At certain times, you may wish to skip deactivation, notably if you are using SVT for insomnia or to help you fall asleep or plan to go to bed after using SVT. In those instances, your brain will drift to sleep and then naturally speed itself back up again upon awakening. This is what we all do when we fall asleep: we pass from fast beta and relaxed alpha into dreamy theta and then dreamless delta brain waves—and vice versa when we wake up.

However, if after using SVT you intend to go back to work, watch the kids, or drive, then deactivate the subconscious. All you need to do is to go back up the way you went down. If you saw yourself walking down 12 steps, then see yourself walking up 12 steps (script below). If you descended an elevator in your mind's eye, then ascend that same elevator. To make sure you're fully awake and alert, look around the room and name 10 things you see, listen to some high-energy music, or do 25 jumping jacks. If you are using an AVE device (see Chapter 6), do a quick beta session to wake you back up.

OPTIONAL RE-ALERT SCRIPT

Now see yourself boarding that elevator. You'll become twice as alert and awake and return back to your everyday, waking state. You'll feel your consciousness returning to your body. That's right.

1. Feel yourself becoming alert now.

2. As you ascend, you're becoming more awake. Your consciousness returning to your body . . . feeling more and more present on every floor.

3. *Perhaps giving a wiggle to your fingers and your toes.*

4. *That's right. Alert and awake.*

5. *Twice as energized and awake as the floor before.*

6. *Riding up another floor.*

7. *Really feel a renewed sense of energy return to your mind and body.*

8. *That's right.*

9. *Alert and activated . . . and wiggling those fingers and toes a bit more now.*

10. *Feeling your body ascend. Consciousness now fully returning to your body.*

11. *Almost there.*

12. *Eyes open. And when they do, you feel completely rejuvenated, rested, and recharged.*

The full script of The 3/12/7 Method, including the re-alert, is part of each audio track. I suggest listening to the audio track for this chapter a few times, even though it does not include SVT steps 3 through 7. It's an easy way to start exercising your subconscious brain. Doing so will allow you to later take SVT to a deeper level with specific concerns or conditions that you want to transform. Now it's time for you and your own subconscious brain to heal your past so you can create a bright and better tomorrow.

CHAPTER 5

Seamless SVT: Adding Steps 3 Through 7

Now that you've experienced what it's like to activate your subconscious brain, you may be surprised to discover that steps 3 through 7 take no extra work. If you listened to the audio or read and visualized The 3/12/7 Method script, you already know what to do: relax, listen, and be open. This part of SVT is where I will incorporate additional cognitive-behavioral techniques, guided visualization, and other tools to supercharge the power of your subconscious.

You don't need to memorize steps 3 through 7 in an analytical way, because the guided audio tracks and scripts with this book will lead you through them in an experiential way. With my patients who are working on a particular issue, I usually suggest practicing SVT at least two times a week on their own for a minor mood boost. For elusive conditions like fibromyalgia or a life-shattering breakup, I suggest they practice SVT daily. The repeated practice helps break long-standing thought patterns and disrupt feedback loops (e.g., depression, pain, the gut–brain axis). Let's take a look at what's happening once you start practicing SVT and begin noticing how your mind creates new thought patterns.

SVT Step 3: Revising the Past

With enhanced access to past memories thanks to those theta brain waves, you'll gain self-awareness and begin to understand yourself in a new way. Some of the SVT scripts accompanying this book will prompt you to revisit memories as if you're pressing the "play" button. If you find any negative experiences there, I'll help you let go of them. By doing so, it's like you're pressing "record" to tape over the distressing memories, or as though you are editing a film where you could turn down the volume and alter the image size to make it small, or blurry, or change it from color to black and white.

Thus, this step has two potential goals. First, in pressing your "play" button, you gain *insight* by understanding the way your past affects the person you are today. This will help you to understand the root of your pitfall thought patterns and negative mantra. Consider someone who struggles with the pitfall thought patterns personalization, pessimism, and paralysis by analysis—and a negative mantra that says, "I'm not good enough." This person may recall the first time these feelings arose, revealing how and why this early experience became pitfall thought patterns and a negative mantra.

If you find anything unpleasant in your past, then you can also benefit from the second goal of this step: reprocessing negative memories using your "delete" and "record" buttons, which are optimized by those theta brain waves. Your subconscious brain can either reframe any negative memories or make them feel less powerful. Instead of focusing on all the ways you felt out of control at the time, you could choose to replay the memory by focusing on what you did control.

Depending on what has happened in your past, SVT gives you the opportunity to revisit the same memory over and over, reprocessing it in different ways and to differing degrees, or to discover a different memory each time you practice SVT for a new condition or concern. It doesn't really matter; what matters is that your subconscious brain knows what is best for you and what you are ready to see.

Or perhaps you believe in a concept that's somewhat similar to Jung's "collective unconscious." If you do, continued practice of SVT may help you unearth an image or archetype of great meaning or spiritual significance. In the early 1900s, Jung distinguished his theory of the "collective unconscious" from Freud's "personal unconscious." The former encompasses the soul of humanity at large, while the latter focuses on one's own personal sexual fantasies and repressed images. Is it possible that you'll tap into a universal archetype like the ones we find in many fables, cultural legends, and myths? Do you personally believe that you can tap into your grandmother's dreams? Or perhaps the narrative your subconscious is weaving about your grandmother's dreams is helping you to make sense of your role in the family, and you know that it's symbolic of what she did for you. Either way, I've had patients who have had deeply healing experiences with SVT. It is not my job to tell you what to believe, but when it comes to brain science, I will say this: if you do believe that you can tap into something greater or more spiritual, SVT would certainly be a method to help you to do so. Many patients I've treated say loved ones have visited them in dreams, or they have had healing, dreamlike visions during SVT. Theta waves are healing, spiritual, and, of course, are the brain waves of dreams.

Remember, SVT is a practice. This means that you can use it over time. You don't have to heal your life all at once. As the subconscious brain knows you're ready to see more, it's possible that it will unlock forgotten or repressed memories. This book is a self-guided version of SVT that is appropriate as a stand-alone or add-on tool for many goals. If the negative memories that you discover are major ones, find a licensed health care professional who is trained in SVT or another protocol effective in processing trauma.

SVT STEP 4: ENHANCING THE PRESENT

Insight and reprocessing helped you move from negative to neutral in step 3. Step 4 will help you move from neutral to positive. You'll use the "play" button again, and you'll examine what's right in your life instead of what went wrong.

See yourself, your identity, and your strengths in a new way. You may find yourself understanding how your past has brought you to the place you are today, and this may help you to reframe any difficulties you've faced as learning experiences. Allow the optimistic and creative subconscious brain to view yourself in a better light. Through SVT, I'll invite you to reexamine your life through a more optimistic, gratitude-centric, and purpose-driven lens. It will be like taking a highlighter to all the times you felt strong, successful, sexy, and smart. In other words, you'll be reminded that you are innately worthy.

Subconscious activation allows access to all the best memories of your life in a way that lets you revisit them as if they're happening in the here and now. This present-moment experience will remind you of the most confident, carefree, jubilant, and joyous times of your life.

This experience can actually *extinguish* your three pitfall thought patterns and negative mantra once and for all. If you are plagued by personalization, when your conscious brain tells you that you didn't get a job because you're not smart enough, your subconscious brain can remind you how brilliant you are—and *show* you the evidence. Following this SVT experience, at some point in your waking life, you will probably be surprised at how different you feel.

The subconscious brain can replace your burden of self-doubt, pessimism, or fear with confidence, optimism, and hope.

The subconscious brain can replace your burden of self-doubt, pessimism, or fear with confidence, optimism, and hope.

Step 4 will help you to receive positive feedback for all the accomplishments you've already achieved. Isn't it interesting that this becomes a rare experience for most adults? Have you ever noticed that our adult world tends to focus more on criticism of what we could be doing better? Won't it be so healing to stop and take time to own your successes and strengths?

SVT's intention is to remind you of your inherent goodness, and each script created for this book includes affirmations of everything you already are. Think about it: We know in raising children that discipline is only truly effective in the long term when rewards outnumber the punishments. This principle doesn't suddenly change just because we are adults; we all need rewards, affirmations, and positive energy. Whether you're 7 or 77, you deserve praise and a pat on the back for all you've accomplished.

The upbeat energy of step 4 helps to create more abundance; negativity blocks this abundance. So we will optimize the present moment so you can be reminded of everything you already are— and of everything that's already *right* with you.

SVT Step 5: Creating the Future

Vividly see your best life unfold step-by-step and day by day with this step as SVT incorporates both guided visualization and cognitive behavioral techniques.

You will look at each daily microtask you need to accomplish to achieve your goals, until it becomes easy for your conscious brain to take over and complete these tasks when you wake up tomorrow. As that occurs, most people quickly notice how they start to feel lighter than air as they rid themselves of past baggage and realize what they are grateful for in their present. Pitfall thought patterns have been extinguished. You probably will already feel a sense of cool, calm, and carefree ease at this point of SVT.

Now you'll have the opportunity to see your future unfold in your mind's eye. Step-by-step, you'll see your best tomorrow. This is the power of cognitive rehearsal, which you'll experience in each SVT script. It will probably feel as if you're actually experiencing your best future right here and right now. With the brain's occipital lobe lit up and a skewed perception of time, 30 seconds of intense visualization feels as though you've already pulled off mind-boggling feats. And if you've already conquered something in your mind's eye, then it's so much easier to do it in the real world. After all, your brain thinks, *I've already done this before.*

For instance, the Olympic diver who practices in her mind's eye may feel like she's actually in that back dive, doing two and a half somersaults in the pike position. Perhaps you'll see everything you'll need to do in the next two and a half years to create the business you've dreamed of.

The power of dissociation—the experience that helps you to feel like you can leave your body for a brief moment—and the distortion of time (both of which were discussed in Chapters 2 and 4) become helpful therapeutic tools during this step. When you see your incredible future unfold, you may also be surprised to find it feels easy and relaxed in your waking, conscious life. When this happens, you're connecting what you see with the help of the subconscious brain with the actions your conscious brain will help you to carry out. In many ways, this connection is the bridge that turns dreams into your reality.

In many ways, this connection is the bridge that turns dreams into your reality.

SVT STEP 6: PLANTING POSITIVITY

Now that you are deep in subconscious activation, with very slow theta brain waves, you are exceptionally open to receive positivity. Without the defenses of the conscious to block positive thoughts, you are more able to absorb them. You may be surprised to notice how often these optimistic beliefs start to bubble up throughout your day.

As you know, delivering suggestions to your subconscious brain while you're in this state can help you achieve amazing goals in your conscious, everyday life. That's thanks to the way the subconscious decreases connections between various parts of your brain. By making you blissfully unaware of your actions, you engage in healthy activities without giving them any thought. This is one of the most gratifying parts of SVT. As discussed in Chapter 2, suggestions delivered to the subconscious unfold in a way that feels so effortless that research subjects reported they felt as though they were "happening as if by an outside force." That's because the messages are operating on a level below conscious awareness.

In fact, you don't even need to consciously take note of every word that's said throughout this journey, because your subconscious is taking all of it in. Your subconscious knows we are setting you up for success. I try to repeat most positive messages at least three times so that they stick in the subconscious brain. These will show up at some point in the future, when you may notice your subconscious helping you pull off some truly fantastic feats with calm, carefree, and confident ease.

SVT Step 7: Building Bridges

Through this book, I'll help you to connect what you're doing in the SVT practice into your waking life by creating a reminder that you can take with you. Your brain pairs experiences, feelings, and our internal chemical responses all the time. You walk into a dark room, and a cat jumps at you—scaring you half to death. Now your brain has paired cats with that creepy dark room and the stress hormone, adrenaline, that was released. Use this phenomenon to your advantage. You could even use it as an antidote to that fear. Create your own inner positivity, and pair it. When you do so, your body and brain will release their stores of feel-good neurotransmitters whenever you'd like. By visualizing a physical "button" on your dominant index finger, you'll be able to access the best parts of what you've discovered here in your SVT

Your brain pairs experiences, feelings, and our internal chemical responses all the time.

practice. You can press this whenever you need to be reminded of your strengths, lovability, and inherent worth in your daily (conscious) life.

Your practice of SVT will also help you let go of anything that's not serving you by visualizing a balloon tied to your nondominant index finger. By rubbing your thumb against your nondominant index finger, you'll be reminded of the light string that's holding that balloon. Instead of helium, you will fill that balloon with all the "hot air" of the naysaying nonsense of the conscious brain. Then, you will use the subconscious brain and the power of your mind's eye to see it float far, far away.

WHAT IT TAKES

All it takes to practice steps 2 through 7 of SVT is your willingness and permission to activate your subconscious brain. As you practice each script, you may not be aware of the changes taking place in your brain—and that doesn't really matter. What's important is the ability of your subconscious to make the changes for you. Perhaps SVT will become your go-to method for healing chronic pain, creating a successful career, transforming relationships, or addressing new triggers for pitfall patterns. Before we dive into transformation of fear, anxiety, mood, insomnia, pain, health, spirituality, and success, I suggest setting aside 30 to 40 minutes at least a few times a week for the next few months. I hope you'll be surprised to discover the wonderful changes that your brain will start creating in your conscious, waking life.

CHAPTER 6

Power Boost SVT

You've now had a mini-experience of what it feels like to tap into the astonishing potential of your subconscious brain. In the next part of this book, I'll help you focus its power like a laser beam as we turn it toward any area in your life that you'd like to master.

First, I'd like to teach you a way to further enhance the activation of your subconscious brain. It's called *audio-visual entrainment*, or AVE.

What is AVE? Decades ago, AVE was clunky and very expensive, and you could only harness its power in a hospital. Today, AVE is a battery-operated, lightweight, wearable, high-tech set of glasses and earphones small enough to carry with you in a purse or a backpack. AVE looks like virtual reality glasses, but the lights and sounds have a more specific goal. If you'd like, you can have the ability to enhance your brain at any time. (If you'd like to see what AVE looks like today, see the modern versions at drmikedow.com.)

AVE has an interesting history that dates back to World War II. Like many of the most potent medical treatments, AVE was discovered by accident. Dr. William Kroger, the physician who helped the FBI in the famous Chowchilla kidnapping case (see page 22), noticed an interesting phenomenon occurring in some military professionals: The slow, sweeping light of the radar screen put some radar operators into a subconscious brain–based trance.

Their brains were synchronizing to the slow lights of the radar screen and sounds of the beeps. If you're in this subconscious brain–based state, you're basically the opposite of alert. That's certainly not great for someone who's monitoring for signs of an invading enemy, is it? But what a wonderful state to experience if you want to relax or recharge.

With this observation, Dr. Kroger teamed up with the Schneider Instrument Company to create a device called the Brain Wave Synchronizer. This early AVE device looked a 1990s boombox. It included a xenon strobe light with dials that controlled the speed of the light. Those lights "synchronized" the brain, with different settings that could help to speed brain waves all the way up to fast beta brain waves, making someone more alert. The slower setting would have mimicked what happened with the radar operators— causing drowsiness.

Dr. Kroger and his colleagues used the Brain Wave Synchronizer to put patients into a dreamy, pain-free state with a theta brain wave setting. It's been said that the device helped produced a deep subconscious state quicker than other technology-free methods. I, too, have found that AVE helps people to quickly and deeply activate their subconscious brains (comparing AVE-enhanced SVT versus SVT without AVE).

Would you be surprised to learn that before the invention of modern pain-relieving medications, the subconscious brain provided pain relief so effective that doctors used it for surgery patients?[1] Dr. Kroger even used the Brain Wave Synchronizer to provide pain relief to women in labor. For women choosing home births or hospital births without an epidural, could AVE-enhanced SVT help? Dr. Kroger thought so.

If that's true, imagine what the subconscious could do to help our modern pain pill epidemic. Recent headlines have shown that even over-the-counter pain relievers such as Advil and Aleve aren't without their risks. The nonsteroidal anti-inflammatory drug you reach for to help achy joints, a sore shoulder, or tension headaches can increase your risk of heart attack or stroke in just the first week of use. This is true for ibuprofen (Motrin, Advil), naproxen (Aleve), and Celebrex. Maybe you think you're doing your body good; after all, it's an anti-inflammatory agent, and you heard that was helpful. But a "strong" 2015 warning from the FDA (they had made a weaker one in 2005) was crystal clear: "NSAIDs can increase the risk of heart attack or stroke in patients *with* or *without* heart disease or risk factors for heart disease." This means everyone is at risk.[2]

Could SVT with AVE be a way to save pain pill–addicted Americans from a life of addiction? Or perhaps it could simply ease some achy joints or an achy shoulder. Would you like to use your subconscious brain to achieve relief and relaxation?

THE BEAUTY OF SYNCHRONIZATION

Believe it or not, you've probably already experienced AVE at some point in your life if you've ever found yourself gazing at a light show set to music or watched swirling fire or glow sticks that were tethered to rope at a luau, drum circle, or electronic dance event. The fire or glow sticks were oscillating to music, and this music was probably in 4/4 time. Remember, that's the musical rhythm of theta waves.

The small, wearable AVE device of today uses the same principle as the Brain Wave Synchronizer. How exactly does this modern version of AVE work in your brain? Well, let's say you put the AVE on the theta brain wave setting and pair it with The 3/12/7 Method. The AVE device then is *entraining*, or synchronizing, your brain waves. Let's unpack this concept.

Picture one of those old, glamorous Hollywood movies featuring synchronized swimmers. Now use your subconscious to help you vividly imagine the trio of swimmers. The first two swimmers—the lights and sounds—are always in perfect unison. The third swimmer is *your brain*. When you put the device on, it's as though your brain is jumping into the pool to join these two old-school, hairpinned beauties. Your brain, though, would be a Lucille Ball–type character who does a cannonball into the pool. At first, Lucille is all over the place. She's definitely *not* in perfect unison. She's probably kicking sporadically and splashing the families watching the show in their tuxes and gowns. In a way, she's an anxious and *conscious* version of your brain.

But then something magical happens: Lucille learns the art of synchronized swimming. Within a few minutes, she falls into line with the other two perfectly poised swimmers. Soon, all three of them are kicking and paddling in perfect unison. Now Lucille is the calm, dreamy, *subconscious* version of your brain. The theta brain wave session is helping your brain "kick and paddle" more slowly.

When you place the AVE on the theta brain wave setting, you'll feel it. Trust me. Just like The 3/12/7 Method—it's a noticeable shift to a calmer, more creative space of wonder. And it means that your subconscious brain is now even *more* deeply activated. Remember: the transition from conscious brain to subconscious means that you're transitioning from beta to theta. And that means that you're transitioning from a state of fight-or-flight (sympathetic nervous system) to rest-and-digest (parasympathetic nervous system). Everything from your immune system to your digestion works better when your parasympathetic nervous system is dominant more often. Less cancer and fewer heart attacks. More healing and health.

WHAT AVE CAN DO FOR YOU

What can today's modern, wearable, at-home version of AVE help you to do? Four things:

1. When placed on the *theta brain wave setting*, AVE can help you dive even deeper into your own subconscious brain. This is the primary reason I recommend AVE. I have found that AVE can help people who have reported difficulty with other subconscious-based practices to enter a deep, wondrous theta state. The

deeper you dive into the subconscious, the more likely it is that the positivity you'll hear in step 6 of SVT will stick. When your subconscious brain receives these suggestions during SVT, it will save them to feed to your conscious brain at some point during your waking life. As SVT changes connectivity in the brain, healthy behaviors begin to "just happen" without thought. Perhaps sooner than you expect, you'll begin to achieve your goals. Would you like to find out how quickly that can happen?

2. When placed on the beta brain wave setting, AVE can help you become more alert. Some brains don't have enough fast beta brain waves and thus have trouble with focus and attention. I wonder if a 10-minute beta brain wave session before completing a project, writing a paper, or getting through your to-do list could help your brain focus without the need for excess caffeine.

3. When placed on the alpha brain wave setting, AVE can help you relax. Meditation is associated with a fairly slow alpha brain wave. People who have practiced mindfulness meditation and hypnosis will recognize elements of both practices in SVT. Those who have previously tried both often say that hypnosis feels deeper than meditation. That's because hypnosis is mostly theta; meditation is mostly alpha. But alpha is still a wonderfully calming brain wave. Doesn't a 10-minute alpha brain wave session sound like a restorative rest after a long day at work?

4. When placed on the delta brain wave setting, AVE can help you fall asleep naturally. As you know, the brain moves from fast to slow brain waves as it's falling asleep—from beta to alpha to theta to delta. Theta is the brain wave of dreams. Delta is the brain wave of deep, dreamless sleep. Restorative sleep should have *both* theta and delta brain waves.

Theta is already present every night when you dream. Isn't it magical that you don't have to wait for dreamtime to call upon this deeply creative state? You can now invite it into your brain whenever you'd like.

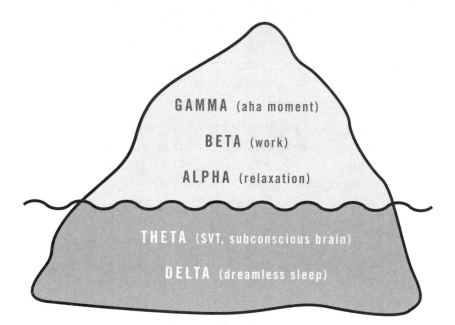

A FEW CONSIDERATIONS

Now, it's important to understand that just as too much beta is *too fast*, too much theta is *too slow*. Excess beta is associated with both PTSD[3] and pain.[4] So if you know that your brain is already too "fast" (e.g., if you suffer from PTSD, pain, or anxiety), then you don't need to use the AVE beta brain wave setting. Use the other, slower settings on the AVE if you're doing a stand-alone session instead.

On the other end of the spectrum, lingering in theta brain waves all day is not healthy. The FDA now recognizes that too much theta and not enough beta is associated with ADHD. In

2013, a brain wave EEG test was approved to help diagnose this disorder.[5] Research even supports beta sessions of AVE as a potential alternative for the Adderall epidemic. Students with brains that need to "speed up" and who used beta brain wave sessions of AVE had decreased inattention and impulsivity and improved reading scores.[6] Thus, anyone with a "sluggish" brain (e.g., those suffering from ADHD-like symptoms, depression, fatigue) can benefit from a beta brain wave session of AVE in the morning or early afternoon. In general, healthy, healed brains should be flexible and experience the right type of brain waves at the right time.

If you experience any of those symptoms, I'll help you to use sessions of AVE-enhanced SVT in the evening to see a happier, healthier you—enhanced with a theta brain wave. Tomorrow morning, you can use a beta brain wave AVE session. And in the afternoon, you may start to notice that all the positivity I gave you last night will start to take flight.

Now, it's been said that both angels and demons "live" in theta. That means that while the vast majority of people will find a blissful, spiritual, and freeing experience in the subconscious, since theta is a dreamlike state where visual memories are stored, dipping down into theta can also mean that unprocessed traumatic memories have the potential to bubble up. If you have severe and untreated trauma, I recommend that you see a licensed health care professional who is also trained in SVT or has experience treating trauma. It can be scary for rape or war survivors to go through this alone. A professional can help "contain" you with advanced methods when these traumatic memories come to mind.

Theta is the brain's best way to take an eraser to painful memories if you truly want to be free of them.

That being said, remember that *theta is the brain's best way to take an eraser to painful memories if you truly want to be free of them.* Just because you aren't consciously aware of the monsters locked in the basement doesn't mean they don't affect you. Medicating with alcohol or treating symptoms with antidepressants or Xanax without SVT isn't ever going to heal the root of the trauma. SVT can address this—especially advanced SVT with a licensed health care professional.

When Not to Use AVE

- Don't use a stimulating beta setting at night, since it can prevent restful sleep.
- If you've ever been diagnosed with bipolar disorder, don't use the beta setting. Theoretically, it could nudge the brain into mania or hypomania.
- AVE should not be used by people with photosensitive epilepsy. If you have ever experienced a seizure triggered by flashing lights, do not use this device. People with epilepsy can use The 3/12/7 Method instead.
- If you have light-sensitive migraines, see if you can tolerate the AVE on the softest light setting. Or you can use the AVE with just earphones and not the glasses. Alternatively, place a tissue in between the glasses and your eyelids to see if you can tolerate a very soft pulse of light.
- If you have a brain injury or severe mental illness, check with your neurologist or other treating health care professional before using AVE.

THAT WONDERFUL FEELING

People often ask what AVE-enhanced SVT feels like. Like SVT itself, it's so powerful that it's hard to explain unless you've experienced it. But let me break down the experience by comparing it to something you have probably felt.

A beta session will make you feel like you had a shot of espresso. *Whoa! Now I'm awake!* An alpha session will make you feel like you've had a cup of chamomile tea. *Feeling a little calmer now. . . .* A theta session will make you feel like you've become transfixed by the most artistic light and sound show you've ever seen. Your body and brain let go of tension and worry. *Oh boy, does my body feel relaxed. And . . . I don't even remember what I was worrying about just before I started this session.* A delta session will make you feel like you've just woken up from a nap or will make you take one. *Zzzz. . .*

So what about The 3/12/7 Method versus AVE? Should I just do SVT on its own, or do I need AVE-enhanced SVT? They each have their own benefits. The 3/12/7 Method is free, whereas AVE requires the purchase of a device. To maximize subconscious brain activation, use The 3/12/7 Method with a theta brain wave session of AVE.

One unique benefit of AVE is that it helps many people who have gone *fairly* deep with The 3/12/7 Method to go even deeper into the subconscious. The more the subconscious brain is activated, the more the ideas suggested to you during SVT are going to stick to your subconscious brain, and the more effortless the behaviors become.

Wouldn't it be so wonderful for an optimistic suggestion planted during a session of SVT to effortlessly grow—like a seedling that suddenly shoots up from the soil? For instance, tonight you may hear during an SVT recording how confident and carefree you'll be in an upcoming work presentation. Then, during tomorrow's presentation, you'll suddenly notice a sense of calmness spreading through your whole body. Where did *that* come from?

Perhaps I'll tell you that every time you see a cigarette or donut, you'll be reminded of a person in your life who made you feel sensationally supported. A thought comes over you: *I got this.* How did *that* get into your brain? You never had *that* thought before. Or you'll become completely blind to triggers. We can even rewire the brain to make donuts taste a bit like a toilet seat if you'd really like to be done with them.

AVE can also be used for other purposes. On the beta, alpha, and delta settings, it's a beneficial, drug-free, stand-alone treatment to aid focus, relaxation, and sleep, respectively. Although you have to *buy* an AVE device, it is a onetime cost. So if AVE replaces a lifetime of medication, it can actually save you money in the long run. More importantly, it can prevent the need for drugs in the first place.

AVE may even help to boost neuroplasticity (your brain's ability to change and reorganize itself), making it an effective long-term strategy for brain health.[7] As you are probably beginning to realize, harnessing the state of your brain can be a potent, natural way to change the way you feel without medication. No wonder so many people feel so relieved and excited to learn of the abilities of the subconscious brain.

USING AVE

The AVE device I recommend on my website has different settings of intensity, so you can maximize or minimize the light and sound. If you are extremely light-sensitive and get headaches or migraines, placing a tissue behind the AVE glasses softens the visual effect. If you are visually challenged, blind, hard of hearing, or deaf, AVE will work with just the sound or the light. However, AVE is more effective if you can use both light *and* sound. Use The 3/12/7 Method simultaneously with the AVE device on the theta brain wave setting to enhance subconscious brain activation. Most people prefer to keep the AVE device on for the entire session. However, some people just like to use the AVE to help them activate their subconscious brains and then prefer to turn the device off at some point during the SVT practice.

There are several ways to use the headphones included with an AVE device and simultaneously hear the SVT audio tracks included with this book. Use external speakers to listen to the SVT audio tracks, and use headphones for the AVE device. Or use two sets of headphones, one for AVE and one for SVT: over-the-ear type for AVE and in-ear type for SVT. You can also just use the glasses from the AVE device without the headphones if you prefer—as a visual entrainment–only option with SVT.

INTERVAL TRAINING YOUR BRAIN

If you are concerned about taking care of your brain, I imagine you also want to take care of your body. If you've read my books *The Brain Fog Fix* or *Heal Your Drained Brain*, you probably already have a deep understanding of how taking care of your body and taking care of your brain go hand in hand—and some practical knowledge about ways you can do so. Both books provide recipes, and they explain how vitamins and amino acids support neurotransmitter production.

The takeaway is that you want your brain, just like your body, to be like an Olympic athlete doing interval training, with short bursts of all-out sprints between low-intensity periods. That type of training helps an athlete's cardiovascular system improve and become flexible. Then the body is capable of handling fast sprints, endurance runs, or anything that's required during a race. By the same token, you want your brain to be able to alternate between sprinting beta brain waves and strolling theta brain waves.

Generally speaking, exercise is a good thing. But if you sprinted for 18 hours a day, that would be bad for your joints. It would actually *accelerate* aging, not prevent it. Sleep is also wonderful. But sleeping too much can also be a bad thing. You don't want to sleep for 4 hours a day, but neither do you want to sleep for 18 hours a day, do you? Eight hours may feel *just right*. The same concept applies to your brain waves. Become a brain waves Goldilocks: not too fast, not too slow, but just right. And like someone who goes to interval training, learn to go up and down. Getting "stuck" at either end of the spectrum can prevent you from reaching your true potential—and reaching your potential is what SVT is all about. If your brain struggles with the transition from beta, through alpha and theta, to delta, you may have trouble falling asleep. If it struggles with the reverse transition, you may have trouble concentrating or getting organized for an important work presentation. The beauty of AVE-enhanced SVT is that you can also use it as an add-on tool to speed up the brain or slow it down, depending on what your brain needs.

When you have to give a presentation at work, wouldn't it be so nice to have your brain sprint? And when you need to be more creative, wouldn't it be magical to call upon the subconscious? That's your brain slowing down to a stroll by generating theta brain waves. That's what SVT enhanced with AVE can do for your brain.

Sooner than you'd ever expect, your brain will become lithe with AVE-enhanced SVT. With the ability to sprint and then stop on a dime, what extraordinary achievements will *your* brain help you to attain?

PART II

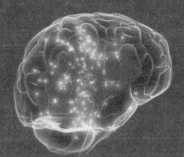

*Putting SVT to
Work for You*

CHAPTER 7

SVT for Letting Go

What goals do you want help with? What psychological, physical, spiritual, or business-related changes do you want to achieve? Most people who learn how to use SVT will put it to use to help them attain a range of incredible achievements—from health to wealth. In this and every chapter that follows, I'll help you put SVT to work by specifically targeting a different goal. After all, SVT is a holistic approach.

Remember, the subconscious has access to parts of the brain that other tools don't. The subconscious brain can regulate pain, digestion, and the immune system—and thus heal and optimize the body. By helping you feel calm and confident, the subconscious may assist you to close multimillion-dollar business deals and handle coaching Little League. If you'd like, the subconscious brain can support your spiritual life. It's been said that theta brain waves are where "the angels" are stored—so you can even use your brain to recharge your soul. The theta brain waves of the subconscious allow you also to access the past so you can make sense of it and let go of anything not serving you. That's what I'll help you do in this chapter.

Spiritual Connections

Want to supercharge your spiritual practice? Whether you connect to the divine through meditation, prayer, religious forms, or other rituals, SVT can deepen your practice and spiritual connections. See the Appendix starting on page 236 for insights and a related SVT practice.

I wonder if your subconscious brain has already started to conspire in your favor. Without your conscious awareness, it probably already knows exactly which goal it would like you to focus on first, second, and so on. Isn't that comforting? We'll begin with letting go, because so often, releasing old patterns, behaviors, thoughts, and emotions is the foundation for other transformation.

WHY LET GO

Letting go is a universal struggle. Relationships go south. Business deals blow up. Unexpected loss takes us for a turn. And when that happens, the volume of the "itty bitty shitty committee" in your conscious brain gets turned up. That "committee" robs you of the cool, calm, carefree confidence you once had. You get stuck in pitfall thought patterns, feelings, and actions that block your long-term potential. Learning to let go—and actually doing it in practice—can feel like a never-ending battle, especially because you typically engage your conscious brain to overcome or transform something from your past that is lodged in your subconscious brain. It's like asking a mathematician to recite Shakespeare.

SVT is so effective because it engages your subconscious to reveal where you're stuck and the memories tied to it. Using SVT is like asking your inner artist to recite that sonnet. Then, SVT helps you reframe the past and create a healthier, happier future. Wouldn't you like to experience the freedom of letting go?

In a few minutes, but not quite yet, we'll officially start the SVT journey of letting go by going back in time. The subconscious brain will hand you the keys to open the doors of your past. If you'd like, you can step into rooms you had completely forgotten about. Or, when you're ready, you might access rooms that had been locked.

Remember how the subconscious takes care of us? You may be surprised to discover that the subconscious also knows when you're ready to see a memory. That's when it grants you access. Memory suppression is part of the subconscious brain's magic. In many ways, your subconscious brain is your inner mother to your inner child.

If your subconscious brain hands you the key to a memory, your slow theta brain waves allow the "play" button in your brain to work better so you are able to see everything in greater, more visceral detail. You may experience sights, sounds, and smells as if they're actually unfolding in the here and now. To truly "reprocess" a memory—and clear it from your brain—this is what you have to do. Don't go around the memory with self-medication or avoidance; go through it.

Some people ask: Why would I want to go back in time? Do I have to reexperience a breakup or business deal gone bad? The answer is yes—if that experience is still bothering you or holding you back in some way. But that's not the only reason. I've often found that patients who don't consciously know a memory is holding them back in some way will discover one once the subconscious brain has a peek at it.

Going back is how you dislodge an emotionally charged memory that is stuck in your brain. Think of it like rebooting your computer if your Internet browser freezes and prevents you from using Word—you obsessing about your ex (the frozen browser) when you should be focusing on work (Word). In this case, you do need to go back to think about that breakup—but just for a few minutes. Then, the supercharged subconscious experience will set you free.

If You Have a Happy Past

Some people ask, "But what if my past was happy? Do I still need this chapter?" Yes. This chapter can help you understand how forgotten memories all fit together—shaping you into the incredible person you are today. Also, isn't it nice to remember our best memories? The subconscious brain isn't about pathology (i.e., telling you what's wrong with you). Your subconscious brain focuses on what's right with you. The subconscious can remind you who you are—and why. It can help you answer the questions: Who am I? What am I here for? How can I put my greatest gifts to use in this world?

The theta brain waves your subconscious brain generates are involved in memory formation and retrieval,[1] and they play a role in modulating emotionally charged memories in traumatized individuals.[2] So we'll also edit those memory files. Here, the subconscious is the program a director uses to stitch expensive scenes together on a computer. Remember when Leonardo DiCaprio and Kate Winslet (two actors we used in other subconscious brain–based metaphors) were in *Titanic* together?

Well, imagine writer/director James Cameron filming these actors on a sound stage. He imagines what he wants them to say. Then, James edits the footage, deciding which scenes stay and which scenes go. They weren't actually on the *Titanic* on the middle of the ocean. But to you, the viewer in that big movie theater, it sure *looks*, *sounds*, and *feels* as though they were, doesn't it? Of course, some part of you *knew* that you were just watching a movie. Another part of you *felt* like you were seeing two people in the middle of the ocean as water poured into a sinking ship.

So now you're James Cameron. Now you write and direct. You decide which scenes stay or go. If you'd like, edit the scenes. Rewrite Leo's dialogue. Jack wouldn't say that to Rose. He'd say this instead . . . Change the filter. Grab some stock footage to make it look as though you've shot the whole thing in Greece if you'd like. Make it look prettier, sunnier. Summertime. Too loud? Turn down the volume. Would you like to see the memory in a more optimistic, strength-oriented, or growth-focused way? Would a different mind-set help you be more productive? Well, did I mention that Oprah is on staff as your head writer? Yep, she's writing your inner dialogue for you. Or you can hire any go-getting guru of your choosing. In fact, you can visualize anything you'd like . . . anything at all. This is your film.

The rational part of you will still know that it didn't unfold in the way that you're editing it. You'll still know where your ex lives or that you didn't close that business deal just as you knew that Leonardo DiCaprio was still alive when you walked out of that movie theater. But the part of your brain that stores sense-based memories, holds on to resentments, or gets sticky with emotion will feel more free.

THE BIOLOGY OF SVT IN LETTING GO

The audio track (and script) for this chapter also incorporates something called bilateral stimulation. This will occur during step 3 of SVT. Bilateral stimulation is simply alternating left-right stimulation on either side of your body. Anything you feel on the right side of your body corresponds with the left side of your brain and vice versa. So on a basic level, the bilateral stimulation of your body activates both sides of your brain.

Notably, SVT is the first technique to formally combine the healing power of the subconscious brain with bilateral stimulation. In my practice, I have used these three modalities to treat trauma: clinical hypnosis alone, bilateral treatment alone,[3] and SVT (which combines elements of those with CBT, visualization, and mindfulness). Not surprisingly, I have found SVT to be the most effective of the three.

As you use the audio tracks included with this book (see page 242), you'll hear a series of left-right audio tones. In the scripts and audio, I'll also gently encourage side-to-side eye flutter during step 3. Interestingly, most people do this spontaneously once their subconscious brains are activated, and it is part of REM sleep. You just need one or the other, so don't worry if your eyes don't flutter. Audio tones are a good "backup" for people with no left-right eye flutter. You may be thinking, *How on earth would alternating left-right–left-right audio tones help me to let go of a bad breakup or business deal gone wrong?* Stay with me for a moment as I dive deeper into this brain science.

If you've been through a bad breakup or business deal, you probably worry or feel anxious. The emotional hub in the brains of people who've been through traumatic events is too active,[4] meaning the emotional and visual memory–based part of your brain is too dominant. This, of course, increases the likelihood that you get stuck in one of the seven pitfall thought patterns you learned about. Perhaps you get stuck in *paralysis by analysis*: you just can't stop worrying, reliving the distressing experience, and it prevents you from moving forward. The rational and verbal part of your brain (left side) is underactive.

As you know, the subconscious generally activates the *right* side of the brain. But the bilateral stimulation is turning up the *left* side. It's interesting to know that when you activate the left side of the brain, it helps to turn down the activity of an overactive right side. EEG research found this is what bilateral stimulation did to patients being treating for PTSD.[5] We're actually *balancing* your brain so you are able to cognitively process and make sense of what you experienced, even if you're not immediately aware of these changes. If you've seen a stereotypical movie about a veteran with PTSD, you saw a man experiencing Vietnam flashbacks, with an unwillingness to verbalize his experience and a tendency toward self-medication with alcohol—that's too much right brain, not enough left brain. Good news: that Vietnam vet—or any trauma survivor experiencing flashbacks or sensory symptoms—has a brain that responds more quickly to subconscious-oriented techniques than the brains of people who don't have these symptoms.[6]

After the brief period of left-brain activation, you can peacefully shift back to right-hemisphere dominance for the remaining steps of SVT. The right hemisphere is wonderful when I help you incorporate elements of guided visualization and cognitive rehearsal to see your future unfold. Once your brain has "deleted" or "edited" the memories from the emotional and sensory parts of your brain, it's easier to move on and move forward. I wonder if you'll notice one other fantastic phenomenon: after bilateral stimulation, your gamma waves increase—yes, to provide more "aha" moments.[7] *That relationship taught me something! That business deal wasn't right for me anyway . . . that's me making a move based on fear.*

So first, with the help of theta brain waves, the subconscious discovers a memory you're ready to access. Then, bilateral stimulation helps you make sense of your experience—by briefly turning up the rational, logical side of the brain. Next, you may realize what you were meant to learn from that bad relationship or business deal gone wrong—with the help of those gamma brain waves. Finally, steps 4 through 7 shift the brain activity back to the right side of the brain as you visualize your best life unfolding.

When you have 30 to 40 minutes, read the instructions for step 1 on the following pages and then listen to the audio track "SVT for Letting Go" (see page 242 for download information). I usually recommend practicing SVT at the end of the day so that you are free to remain in a relaxed state of mind or even fall asleep after the practice. If you use SVT during the day, then use the optional re-alert followed by a few jumping jacks, wiggle your fingers and toes, and take a walk a few times around the block before driving.

SVT FOR LETTING GO

As a brief review, SVT involves seven steps, most of which only require your permission and participation. You'll do step 1 again now, as it specifically relates to letting go. Then, steps 2 through 7 will happen as one seamless practice within the audio track. I've included the script for letting go as a blueprint for people training in SVT or for you to memorize down the road, when you may be ready to customize your own SVT practice.

- Step 1: Considering the Conscious

- Step 2: Activating the Subconscious

- Step 3: Revising the Past

- Step 4: Enhancing the Present

- Step 5: Creating the Future

- Step 6: Planting Positivity

- Step 7: Building Bridges

LET GO AS OFTEN AS YOU NEED

Any time you find yourself stuck or revisiting pitfall thought patterns, practice this SVT script to reengage your subconscious brain and further embed changes into your conscious, waking life. In fact, the more you activate your subconscious brain, the more it will help your conscious brain act on these changes. Since this SVT for letting go is foundational for many deep-seated issues, I suggest using this practice at least two times this week and coming back to it any time you experience a new trigger. Within just two weeks, you may notice freedom from the pitfall patterns that once held you captive. As your life continues to change, there will be new stressors to release. As an experienced practitioner of SVT, you'll become more adept at letting negativity go quickly. Isn't that nice to know? Like meditation, SVT shifts brain and body from fight-or-flight to rest-and-digest. Thus, practicing it on a regular basis also has general health benefits. I've included the script for letting go as a blueprint for practitioners training in SVT and for people who want to memorize the SVT script so they can practice it without the guided audio tracks.

STEP 1: CONSIDER THE CONSCIOUS

In Chapter 3, you wrote down the three pitfall thought patterns that hold you back the most. Now go back to those thought patterns (page 47). As it relates to a situation you want to move on from, which one pitfall or negative mantra holds you back the most? (Refer back to page 48.) Write it down here:

Type of pitfall thought pattern: _____ which, to me, is a

_____

thought that sounds something like: _____

_____

Now that your conscious brain knows what it needs to change, allow your powerful subconscious brain to figure out how it will change it.

STEPS 2 THROUGH 7 OF SVT FOR LETTING GO

Reminder: you are the observer of everything that unfolds here. So remind yourself that it's okay to use this technique bit by bit. The subconscious brain will deliver only what you're ready to see. The subconscious always has the power to turn down the volume or minimize the size of anything it helps you to visualize.

When you access memories, they can feel lifelike, but the subconscious in its never-ending mission to look out for your best interests will know if it needs to distance you from anything you see, hear, and experience here. Isn't it so nice to know you always have the power to ground yourself as the observer of this healing process? You also have the power to mute the "film," minimize the screen, or close the scene altogether at any time. Isn't it nice to know that you're in control at all times? Remember, your subconscious is responsible for your gut feelings and intuition, so it has a deep sense of what's right for you.

Now find a comfortable, seated position. Being relaxed makes this process easier and deeper. If SVT makes you sleepy, then you'll easily fall asleep later. For your initial practice, listening to the audio track "SVT for Letting Go" is the easiest way to get started (see page 242).

I invite you to begin by simply allowing the eyes to close as you settle into this safe and serene healing space. And as you settle here into this comfortable state of deep relaxation, I wonder which part of your body feels most relaxed.

You already know how to activate the subconscious brain . . . and we'll walk through it again in just a moment. Allow our journey to begin now with a bit of mindfulness. Invite yourself— without any sort of judgment—to simply notice what's on your mind . . . right here and right now. Isn't it so interesting that when you can watch your thoughts in this particular way? It may even feel relaxing and restorative. Watching your thoughts is a great place to start your journey of letting go.

*Now gently pivot your attention to sounds . . . as you invite the ears to notice **three sounds** you're hearing right here and right now. That's right. It could be comforting to begin with the loudest sound you can perceive in this moment. Now find a noise that's neither loud nor soft. Now, I wonder what is the faintest sound you can hear . . . Can you hear your breath? That's right. Perfect.*

*Now invite the eyes to notice **two colors** you can see . . . even with the eyelids closed. The first being directly in front of you . . . and then, on the next inhale, what color can you see near the crown of the head as you roll the eyes up, up, up?*

*On the next exhale, allow the eyes to float down, down, down . . . now allowing the eyes to just relax as any lingering tightness just floats away. Yes, that's right. And now I invite you to really feel **one breath**. Allowing the breath to breathe you. Can you feel the breath rocking you? Can you feel the place where the breath feels the most pleasant or the most peaceful? Allow that feel-good or soothing sensation to spread through the brain and body. That's right. Perfect.*

As you tune in to your senses in this present moment, you will probably find that the judgment, scrutiny, and defenses of the conscious begin to float away. And you are reminded that the subconscious is always looking out for you; it sees your greatest potential today and what possibilities you can look forward to tomorrow. Throughout this healing journey, you will probably find that images and memories are more vivid and lifelike when viewing them through the lens of the subconscious. I invite you to send a message to the subconscious right now that today, you're only going to see, hear, and experience what you're ready to see, hear, and experience. Call upon the subconscious right now, and softly ask it to help you in the way you most need today. Isn't it so nice to know your subconscious is conspiring in your favor and always knows what you need to heal and grow?

*You have a sense coming to you now that this journey will be a safe and healing one. Visualize **12 steps** in front of you. Perfect. When you take a step, you may notice a sense that the body is actually descending. When that happens, then you'll also notice the mind becoming more and more relaxed. Now I invite you to take a step down. That's right.*

12. *Which foot is taking the first step? Is it the left foot . . . or is it the right? As you feel the body moving down, simply notice a small—or maybe a larger—sense of deep relaxation washing over you. That's right.*

11. *Feeling the other foot take that next step on the staircase now. Allowing this deep relaxation to heal your mind . . . or relax your body.*

10. *Simply allow the body to take all the time it needs. Many people notice the breath becoming slower and more relaxed here. I wonder if you may notice your breath moving down into your belly as it does when the subconscious begins to take over. That's an indication that you're more relaxed. As the breath slows, the mind calms.*

9. *The other foot is taking that next step now, and I wonder if you can actually feel a sense of the body moving down. And as you do, you're becoming so carefree, calm, and comfortable.*

8. *Perhaps sooner than you'd expect, you're noticing now how this relaxation may help you to let go of any tightness in your body. And as that happens, your mind can easily let go of any remnants of conscious thought or worry. That's right. Good.*

7. *Even deeper now. It's almost as if every step down the staircase can help you to become two or even three times more relaxed and rested than you were on the step before. And when that happens, I wonder if you'll just notice how refreshing it all feels. Perfect.*

6. *Halfway down the stairway now. That's right. Letting go a bit more now. Isn't that such a calming feeling? You deserve this rest. You do so much in your everyday life, don't you? Nothing to bother you, nothing to do.*

5. *Almost there now, and you may notice that the mind embodies the same easy "rag doll" quality as you may feel now in the body. It no longer has to do anything. I don't know if you have already begun to feel as though there's something here you were meant to find or if you will find that a bit later. Either way, it can be so incredible just to have this time to rest, relax, and recharge.*

4. *Feeling the next foot take the next step down, and you may notice a wonderful dreamlike state come to you—now or at some point along this journey. And you have a sense that everything you're going to experience here is going to be so healing. Isn't that nice to know?*

3. *Almost there now. That's right. You're doing so wonderfully already . . . and you've only just begun.*

2. *Next-to-last step. Perfect. Feeling twice or maybe even three times as calm, dreamy, or relaxed on this step as you were on the step before.*

1. *Noticing now . . . where the relaxation has spread in brain and body. Just take all the time you'd like here to enjoy this type of experience you're feeling now. That's right. Very good.*

Now that you've felt the body make its way down the staircase, you've probably noticed the brain begin to slow itself down into a state of healing relaxation.

In just a moment, you'll feel the body start to float upward as your consciousness begins to expand and I count up from one to seven. As these two things happen—body floating and consciousness expanding—you may notice an even deeper sense of peace and relaxation.

As the body floats, many people also notice it feels warm as though you're taking a warm bath or floating in the ocean on a summer day. As you practice this more, you may even find that you lose a sense of time and space. You may even find that— if you'd like—you can create a sense of "leaving" the physical body for this healing time you've given yourself. If it feels comfortable, you may wish to see your consciousness actually leaving the physical body as a momentary "out-of-body" experience. Your consciousness will return effortlessly and easily by the time you finish this practice. In fact, you'll be more present than you were before.

Counting now:

1. *Body float.*

2. *Consciousness moving upward and expanding so that it's now larger than the body.*

3. *Body becoming lighter and warmer.*

4. *Consciousness moving upward and expanding even more so that it fills the room.*

5. *Body becoming almost weightless now.*

6. *Consciousness elevated and expanded that it's joining with the universe.*

7. *So deep and so relaxed. Perfect.*

Now I invite you to ask your subconscious to help you by giving you a person or a scene that will help you feel safe . . . and loved . . . and comfortable. I wonder if this person or energy is a companion you'd like to take with you on this healing journey.

If it's a person, you may wish to see him or her next to you. Would you like to see this person taking your hand? It's so nice to know you're not alone, and it's so comforting to know that you're in control. That's right. If you see a feeling or a kind of energy in your mind's eye, perhaps you can feel yourself taking some part of this and stitching it around the heart or stuffing a bit of it in a pocket. That's right. Perfect.

Now that you have your companion, let's open up that editing software. In just a moment, but not quite yet, the subconscious brain will press the rewind button. Ask the subconscious brain to show you a scene that you need to see from your past. You can rewind to a scene itself and, if needed, float all the way back to the first time you felt this way. I'd imagine this will help you ignite a flash of insight—that "aha" moment. And gently notice how these feelings are linked to that pitfall thought pattern.

If it's something simple like a fender bender you'd rather forget, then just go back to the scene itself. But oftentimes, there's something deeper . . . that's why situations affect us so deeply. If you feel like you're being abandoned in your relationship, when was the first time you felt this way? If a business deal went bad and you were reactive, I wonder if there was something in your past that could help you understand why. Does business mean stability to you—and did you need to create stability because your childhood was so instable? Or perhaps there was something about the person you were doing business with who reminded you of someone, and you weren't conscious of it. Or, perhaps, you need to discover something about yourself. I don't know what you'll discover. I know that your subconscious is inherently wise. You already know that, don't you? And as you connect these dots, it will probably bring insight and awareness to the way these deeper links are related to pessimism or paralysis by analysis . . . or any other pitfall thought pattern that prevents you from attaining your healthiest, happiest, and highest self.

First, the subconscious will help you find and mark this scene. In a few moments, but not quite yet, you'll use some of the other buttons in that editing software you have—thanks to your subconscious brain.

Now press that rewind button with your subconscious brain. That's right . . . taking all the time you need . . . floating back in time now . . . yesterday . . . last week . . . last year . . . two years . . . two decades. Going back as far as you need to go . . . to the first time you felt stuck or sad or reactive or resentful. The scene you were meant to see today . . . the one you want to let go of . . . or one that will provide insight so you can see things in a new way. That's right. Did you find the scene?

All I want you to do now is to mark the scene as an editor of a Hollywood film would do. Mark the start of that scene, and mark the end. The scene could be 30 seconds . . . or if you'd like, it could be a montage of scenes that you put together into one short scene.

Before you play that scene, I want you to consider what you are feeling in the eyes. You may have felt something that tends to happen to almost everyone's eyes when they activate their sub-conscious brains. You may not be able to feel it, but if I were in the room with you right now, sitting across from you, I would probably be able to see it. Did you feel your eyes flutter back and forth as you activated your subconscious brain?

As I count backward from three to one, I wonder if the eyes will release just a bit more now. Let's try it now: three . . . two . . . one. Did you feel anything? Now just relax, and every time you press play or use the editing suite in your subconscious brain, I'll invite you to flutter the eyes back and forth—left to right— in that way.

In just a moment, but not quite yet, you're going to press play on the scene you've marked as you invite the eyes to flutter back and forth. If you reach the end of the scene, you can just put it on a loop and begin the scene again. At the same time, you'll also hear tones in your left and right ears. All you need to do this time is to play the scene again. You'll have a chance to edit it in just a minute. Remember: scenes played through the lens of the subconscious brain feel real, but remember that you are the observer of this scene. If it feels too powerful, you can always turn down the volume or minimize or close the screen just as you would do on a computer.

Now press play and invite the eyes to flutter on three . . . two . . . one [left-right-left-right audio tones].

Now inhale on the count of three: one, two, three. Exhale on the count of six: one, two, three, four, five, six. Many people notice tension, but at least one or two places in the body feel at ease. Now, as I count from one to five, the subconscious brain will spread that ease to the rest of the mind, body, and spirit: one, two, three, four, five. That's right. Perfect.

In just a moment, I'm going to have you play that scene again. This time, you're going to see a split screen.[8] *On the left, you'll see the same scene you just saw. On the right side of the screen, the subconscious brain is going to highlight something the conscious brain may have missed: what you already did right in that scene.*

Most of us are so hard on ourselves all the time. So let's allow this generous and kind subconscious brain to highlight what you already did right that day or on those days. If you can see what you've done right, then you can see that your healing has already begun. If you were reactive with a business partner, see all the times you walked away and kept your cool. If felt abandoned in that relationship, see all the times you took good care of yourself in healthy ways. If you did anything to help yourself, zoom in on those parts of the scene on the right side of the screen. Pan to the parts of this scene you'd like to pay attention to.

Now, pressing play with that split screen, see the scene unfold in the split screen, with the left screen showing the scene as you saw it a moment ago and the right screen showing what you did right. If you get to the end of the scene, just begin it again. Allow the eyes to flutter. Now, on three . . . two . . . one . . . [left-right-left-right audio tones].

Now inhale on the count of three: one, two, three. Exhale on the count of six: one, two, three, four, five, six. Many people notice there may be tension, but at least one or two places in the body feel at ease. Now, as I count from one to five, the subconscious brain will spread that ease to the rest of the mind, body, and spirit: one, two, three, four, five. That's right. Perfect.

Now let go of the split screen. This time, your subconscious brain is going to give you access to all the fancy buttons you'd pay extra for on one of those fancy editing programs. It's time to open up that editing software. You're that Hollywood director now. I wonder how the subconscious brain would like to change that scene. Would you like to turn the volume down? Would you like to create a different ending? Perhaps it would be nice to see all the things you did right. I wonder if you could shrink it or put a black-and-white filter on it. Was there something left unsaid—something you would like to say? Isn't it nice to know that you have an opportunity to finish your unfinished business? You probably don't have to think too hard, because your subconscious brain already knows exactly what it needs to do here. Use the creativity of the subconscious to do anything you'd like. In just a moment, the power of the subconscious brain will start to set you free.

This time, play the scene and allow the subconscious to edit the scene in any way it likes. Press delete, press re-record, adjust the volume, or do anything else you'd like. Again, allow the eyes to flutter side to side now in three . . . two . . . one . . . [left-right-left-right audio tones].

Now inhale on the count of three: one, two, three. Exhale on the count of six: one, two, three, four, five, six. Many people notice there may be tension, but at least one or two places in the body feel at ease. Now as I count from one to five, the subconscious brain will spread that ease to the rest of the mind, body, and spirit: one, two, three, four, five. That's right. Perfect.

Now, with gratitude for helping you to "unstick" that stuck memory or behavior from your past, allow the subconscious brain to fast-forward to present day. Now your subconscious brain is helping you to enhance your present life. You're right here. Right now. Present day. I wonder how seeing your past in a new way will help you to see your present in a new and more optimistic light.

As you now consider your life and that present situation you may have been struggling with before, allow your subconscious brain to consider it again. Isn't it so interesting that the subconscious brain has the power to look at things with a sense of what's right? Since you just let go of something that was holding you back, take a moment to notice what feels different now. I don't know if the difference will be a subtle one or a significant one, but you will—at some point—notice something.

Isn't it interesting that in this moment, you may even be able to find one or two pieces of evidence that you are stronger than you realize? After all, people eventually find themselves growing in some way after difficult experiences, don't they? So now the subconscious helps you notice everything that's right with your life. Perhaps it will surprise you that the subconscious is helping you consider your present life through a strength- and growth-oriented lens.

I wonder how everything you've been through has made you into the inherently worthy, wonderful, and wise person you are right here and right now? Isn't that so rewarding to stop and consider? Now consider that pitfall thought pattern you wrote down in step 1. I wonder what part of this experience has loosened the belief. Has the subconscious transformed that negativity into optimism? Does 10 percent or 20 percent or perhaps even 80 percent of you now believe something better for yourself? As you reflect on all this positivity, ask your subconscious to help you write a positive mantra. I wonder if it sounds something like: "I'm okay." "I'm innately worthy." Or "I'm lovable." "I'm confident, gracious, and forgiving." Or "My life is filled with divine purpose." You may find your positive mantra instantly, or it may take you a few moments. When you do find it, you'll probably start to feel a bit more peaceful—or maybe a lot more peaceful. And with more peace comes the ability to cultivate more pleasure. That's right. Perfect. Allow this positive energy to wash over you and all the cells in your brain and body. Yes, you are already so innately lovable and worthy. Remember your strengths and what makes you who you are . . . and why you're here. And perhaps there is even a newfound hope for the future . . . as your yesterday is a little rosier and your present feels a little brighter. In this moment, feel the part of you that is most lovable. I wonder if it's your kindness. Or perhaps your loving heart? Is it your compassion and grace? Are you proud of your strength? Whatever you find here, simply see it as an energy. See yourself and the way you manifest and use this strength in your day-to-day life. That's right. Isn't it so incredible to give yourself credit for that? Perfect. If this strength had a place in your body, where would it be located? Now imagine that you had a dial for your inner sense of strength, and as I count from one to five, you're turning that dial up: one, two, three, four . . . five. That's right. Perfect.

Now the subconscious is going to help you to fast-forward your life and use the power of rehearsal. Many people will notice that an everyday feeling of time begins to float away so that everything you see unfold here in a matter of seconds may actually feel as if you're living it over the course of hours. If you'd like, you could see the next incredible decade of your life unfolding in a minute. Would you be willing to experience and see—in great detail—everything you'd like to create, every word you'd like to communicate, and every change you'd like to make? In fact, you can rehearse anything and everything that will be different in your incredible future. See the specific, measurable, achievable, relevant, and time-sensitive goals unfolding. That's right. . . . You can see it, can't you?

Isn't it incredible that you're now connecting what you feel in this practice with everyday actions? See the microtasks you need to undertake to help your dreams unfold. Do you see them? That's right. Perfect. Step-by-step and day by day. . . . And isn't it so fascinating that the subconscious can help you see it all so vividly? And if you can see it happening, then the subconscious will effortlessly send messages to the conscious in your waking life. That's right. Seeing it all so clearly now.

Now deepen one more time so the positive messages you're about to hear will be planted deep into the subconscious brain. Deepening as I count backward from three to one: three . . . two . . . one . . . that's right. You have done so much here to take care of yourself today, haven't you? Aligning yourself only with the parts of you that are in your best interests. Those parts are your highest self, aren't they? I wonder if it will be tomorrow or if it will be sometime next Tuesday afternoon when you notice that something has changed. You are already a bit more free from your past, aren't you? It's such a pleasant feeling, isn't it? Check in now with your brain and body to see what has lifted . . . and just notice . . . what is already helping and what will continue to help you feel liberated from a memory or an image that was blocking your true potential and truest self. This will become more noticeable tomorrow . . . and the day after . . . and the day after that. I wonder when you will truly notice the pinnacle moment of what it truly means to be set free. Will you feel it in your thoughts, or will it be a change in the way you feel? It will be so wonderful when that pops up. I wonder if you'll enjoy the calm, confident you that begins to show up in a new way . . . each and every day, perhaps sooner than you expect. Whether you're in your office or your home or out in the world, in all probability you'll have a freedom in the way you show up, in the way that you walk . . . because you have changed something, haven't you? Yes, this empowering sense of freedom has already been planted . . . because you planted it. Now I wonder at what day and what time you'll see that first sprout, evidenced by a bloom.

You have probably gained so many insights that have helped set you free. So now, let's build a bridge that will help you connect everything you have done here during this practice—so that you can take it with you into your waking life.

First, what are three of the best things you've gained here? Perhaps they were lessons or insights. I wonder if they were energies or feelings; you could even visualize them as colors if you'd like. Now send the best part of what you've gained down your dominant arm into your dominant hand. Gather and intensify the positivity, freedom, and strength in your dominant index finger. That's right. Now rub the tip of that index finger with that thumb. Can you feel that? There. You've just built a button for yourself. In your waking, everyday life, whenever you need a little piece of what you've created here, all you need to do is to push that button. All the feelings, lessons, or freedom will come flooding back. Feel-good chemicals will flood your brain and body. Isn't it so nice to know this button is here for you at any time?

Second, gather any residual stuff you'd like to get rid of: resentments, negativity, pitfall thought patterns, a feeling of being stuck. Now visualize a balloon tied to your nondominant index finger. Can you feel it? See that balloon being blown up as you fill it with the "hot air" of things that are not in your best interests. Many people may even notice that this finger will begin to lift on its own. Isn't that interesting? One last moment here . . . is there anything else you'd like to put in that balloon? That's right. Now rub that thumb against your nondominant index finger to untie that balloon. In your mind's eye, see that balloon float far, far away. Can you see it becoming so small? Tiny now. Follow it until it's gone. And whenever you notice any of this "stuff" that's not serving you, all you need to do is put it into this balloon that's tied to your nondominant index finger. Then rub your thumb to untie the string . . . and let it all go. You're free.

OPTIONAL RE-ALERT

1. *Feel yourself becoming alert now as you see yourself walking back up those stairs.*

2. *As you walk up another step, you're becoming more awake. Noticing your consciousness returning back into your body.*

3. *Perhaps giving a wiggle to your fingers and your toes . . . as you feel yourself moving up that staircase.*

4. *That's right. Alert and activated.*

5. *Twice as energized as the floor before.*

6. *Feeling yourself in your body, and as you do, feel recharged with a new kind of excitement.*

7. *Up and alert, alert and awake. That's right.*

8. *Renewed, recharged, and reinvigorated.*

9. *Alert and activated . . . wiggling those fingers and toes a bit more now.*

10. *Feeling your body ascend . . . and feeling your consciousness completely back in your body now.*

11. *Almost there.*

12. *Eyes open. And when they do, feel completely rejuvenated, rested, and recharged.*

CHAPTER 8

SVT to Stress Less and Conquer Fears

For some reason, there is a myth that even some professionals in my field still believe: that only cognitive behavioral therapy (CBT) works in conquering phobias and stress. Did you know that your subconscious works just as well? Your subconscious brain can transform your fear and stress. An investigation of 18 controlled clinical trials of generalized anxiety, phobias, and other anxiety disorders found that subconscious brain–based techniques effectively treated these issues and were just as effective as CBT.[1]

So what happens when you put the subconscious brain and CBT together? The answer: the subconscious supercharges good old-fashioned CBT. As you already know, SVT begins by considering the conscious in step 1 and then activates the subconscious in step 2. By combining the power of the two, SVT helps most people work wonders when it comes to conquering fears and stressing less.

THE HEROES YOU NEED

Let's consider this in terms of a superhero movie—also known as your brain conquering fear and stress. CBT is like Superman. Traditional, tried and true, an uncomplicated (stereotypically male) superhero saving the world. University hospitals love this straightforward and easy-to-understand (some would argue dry) method.

Your subconscious is like Natasha Romanoff, the Black Widow, played by Scarlett Johansson. She's complex, a woman who doesn't need saving by some muscle-bound man. In fact, she can take care of herself, thank you very much. Her reputation, like that of subconscious-based methods, is a bit . . . colorful. Some would even say controversial. People don't know what to think about her. Where is she from? What's she about? Can you trust her? She's so mysterious.

The good news: you don't have to choose Superman or Natasha. Both superheroes can help you conquer your fears and stress less. Let Superman (your conscious) and Natasha (your subconscious) work together. They'll accomplish far more as a team.

I wonder what hurdle in your brain they will help you overcome. Would you like to overcome that fear of cats? Would you like to look forward to getting on that plane? Superman and Natasha will have your back. In fact, those two superheroes live inside your brain. They are part of you. Isn't that comforting?

If stressing less sounds nice, Natasha can turn your boss's voice (the one that sends you into sheer dread) into a cue for your body to relax. When you notice it happening, you may think, *That's strange. How did the subconscious transform that voice into a reminder of my own inner well of patience and grace—and send it through my whole body?*

You see, Natasha knows how to access your brain's inner pharmacy of feel-good brain chemicals. Xanax and Paxil aren't the only way to make more GABA (a relaxer) and serotonin (a mood booster) in your brain. If you'd like, the subconscious can flood you with those feel-good chemicals whenever you want—without the side effects of prescription medication. Now, aren't you so glad Natasha is on your team?

THE BIOLOGY OF STRESS AND FEAR

When it comes to reducing stress and conquering your fears, Superman and Natasha are rescuing you from an overactive amygdala. This part of the brain is what noted stress researcher Dr. Bessel van der Kolk calls the brain's "smoke detector." The amygdala, part of your emotional center, alerts you of danger, whether real or perceived. In stress-, anxiety-, and phobia-prone brains, that smoke detector doesn't go off just when there is a fire. It goes off every time you put a piece of bread in the toaster. It's way too sensitive. You once burned a piece of toast, filling your kitchen with smoke and scaring your neighbors. Now any piece of toast is clearly a fire hazard. The result: high stress hormones, panic attacks, and fears. If you've read my book *Heal Your Drained Brain*, you understand this also spikes your risk for heart attack, stroke, and high blood pressure. You also know the integrative strate gies that I recommend to stress less and conquer phobias, such as stress-relieving foods and testing your neurotransmitter levels to determine why you have so much stress or fear in the first place. (For more on this, go to drmikedow.com or my Facebook page.) I'll address this more in other chapters, but combining these with SVT supercharges those practices.

We'll use an SVT script that incorporates the best of conscious and subconscious techniques to turn down the sensitivity of your overactive amygdala. I've helped hundreds of people do this with CBT in my private practice. Traditional CBT would use exposure therapy, taking baby step by baby step: 1) imagine a cat; 2) see a photo of a cat; 3) see a real cat, and so on. I would help you to breathe with each experience, and your amygdala would eventually stop going off all the time. This process is certainly not fun, and it takes a long time. It's wonderful to discover how much more quickly and easily the process goes when you supercharge similar techniques with the subconscious.

One study divided people who were recently exposed to high levels of stress into three groups. Group A got supportive counseling. Group B got good old-fashioned, tried-and-true CBT. Group C got CBT infused with hypnosis. At the end of six sessions, group C had improved the most.[2] An investigation of 18 studies came to a similar conclusion: subconscious brain–enhanced CBT is superior to CBT by itself.[3]

Another incredible biological change that only the subconscious brain can accomplish relates to how we interpret information. Your five senses send information to your brain right here and right now—the bottom-up information. You see a cat, and your eyes send that data to your visual cortex. Then, your visual cortex sends it up the chain. Pieces of information about this object, its color, and its shape are moving up through the brain. At the same time, your brain is filtering sensory data through its database of knowledge derived from experience. This top-down processing creates the framework and filter for how you interpret that bottom-up information. Object, color, and shape come in (bottom-up). And you learned what a cat was when you were a child (top-down). You could say consciousness is what happens when these two signals collide in the brain. At that moment of impact, you say to yourself: *Aha! That's a striped tabby cat.*

However, if your amygdala has stored a stressful memory or emotion about a cat, then your top-down processing may lead you to see a dangerous lion ready to pounce and claw you to death. As *The New York Times* writer Sandra Blakeslee puts it, "What you see is not always what you get, because what you see depends on a framework built by experience that stands ready to interpret the raw information."[4]

Here's the magic of the subconscious brain: it has the power to change top-down processing as it relates to stress and fear. Via top-down processing, the subconscious brain can help you *unlearn* what a cat is. As you know, the brain will just ignore bottom-up information that it doesn't recognize. You see, it has too much information coming in from the outside world to pay attention to everything. Emotional charge helps the brain to file memories or discard them as irrelevant. Case in point: Do you remember where you were on 9/11/2001? Now, do you remember what you ate for breakfast two Mondays ago? So while certain memories or images (e.g., 9/11, that cat you fear) are etched deeply, others are discarded. Remember: the brain is sorting, and it's giving priority to the things it thinks could hurt you. Your subconscious brain is so powerful that, if you learn to harness this unique power through SVT, it can help you ignore anything that's not serving you.

You can also affect the brain in more subtle ways in SVT. Instead of just making objects disappear, tinker with them. In a subconscious brain–activated state, you hear, *Squares are always red.* Later, I show you a blue square. A minute later, I ask you: *What color was that square?* Many people will say *red.* Now, who cares what color a square is? But, I wonder if you'd like to believe *cats are always cute and cuddly creatures or planes are safe and serene or the sound of jet engines is reminiscent of your sweet mother's voice.* Are you starting to understand how tinkering with these processes can help with fear?

When we activate your subconscious, it can also create all sorts of illusions, and SVT can help you to use those illusions to work in your favor. So if you believe or expect cats to be serene and comforting, then when your eyes see a cat, your brain will interpret data differently. That's what that study I told you about in Chapter 2 did. Subjects in the study were told, "Very soon you will be playing a computer game inside a brain scanner. Every time you hear my voice over the intercom, you will immediately realize that meaningless symbols are going to appear in the middle of the screen. They will feel like characters in a foreign language that you do not know, and you will not attempt to attribute any meaning to them."[5]

The subjects didn't play the game inside the brain scanner until days later. That means that the subconscious suggestions that had been planted had stuck. Sure enough, the subjects reacted as if they didn't know how to read English. The Stroop test and a brain scan verified the magic (science) of the subconscious brain. And if the suggestions of not being able to read English could stick for days in these subjects' brains, imagine how SVT could help you deal with stress and phobias in ways that few other methods can.

Wouldn't it be calming to tinker with top-down processing in your brain just like the subjects in that study? Perhaps you'd like not to notice cats at all; why couldn't they be totally invisible to you? Or maybe you have a boss who's not winning any awards for manager of the year. In fact, maybe she reminds you of Miranda Priestly in *The Devil Wears Prada*. Yet you need to hold on to this job for the health insurance. Wouldn't it be nice if I could program your brain—by targeting top-down processing—to believe that any mean-spirited comments would be like a foreign language you couldn't understand? Or we could choose to give you selective amnesia so that you only remember the messages you need to hear from her but you instantly forget all her nasty comments. If it's a fear of planes that stresses you every time you travel, would you like to acquire selective hearing loss so that the roar of the jet engines is simply background noise that you barely notice?

SVT functions like a sort of virtual reality. It tricks the brain into thinking it has already done that thing it feared.

You already know how the subconscious can distort reality and memories. The SVT in this chapter will activate the subconscious brain and then prompt it to imagine you are with that cat or flying on that plane—and it felt as if it were actually happening. When you have a subconscious experience that feels real, the brain (and its amygdala) says, "Oh, I guess can do this." SVT functions like a sort of virtual reality. It tricks the brain into thinking it has already done that thing it feared. SVT also integrates breath techniques by gently encouraging diaphragmatic and exhalation-dominant breathing during visualization, which teaches the brain it can be calm while it "sees" a cat or "hears" a jet engine.

COOL, COLLECTED, CAREFREE

Imagine for just a moment that I planted positivity deep in your subconscious to conquer fears and reduce stress. Would this healing journey be easier for you if I suggested it was so?

Wouldn't it also be interesting if I suggested that the subconscious will continue to work on these issues for you? Interestingly, people who practice SVT regularly often report that the healing continues in their dreams—the playground of the subconscious. You need not give it any conscious effort at all.

Help for Sleeplessness

Is sleeplessness at the root of your stress? Or vice versa? Turn to the Appendix (page 223) for insights and a bonus SVT practice specifically to help you get enough restful shut-eye.

If you'd like, you could even take this to the next level. At some point, it would be enlightening to activate your subconscious and then, when you're ready, the eyes to drift open and gaze at a tablet that has a series of YouTube cat videos ready to go. Or put on a pair of glasses that turn your phone into a virtual reality device and do the same thing. Of course, you can also wear the glasses that come with an AVE device and see the cats with the power of your mind's eye. The beauty of conjuring up your own visuals is that only you know exactly what that cat looked like when you were seven years old at your aunt's house, so only you can shrink that same terrifying cat with the terrible stripes into a tiny and timid kitty with the power of the subconscious. This subconsciously supercharged experience feels amazingly trippy . . . and, by the way, sort of easy. When it's all over, you will have tricked your brain into thinking that you've spent a full day with 100 cats. And at some point in the future, when that real cat wanders into your life, you may not even notice it's there, or maybe you'll feel a sense of calmness wash over you.

Perhaps the subconscious will decide to slowly continue the exposure therapy in your dreams . . . and I wonder if cats will begin to transform into kind and lovable creatures. Who wants to go to more hours of therapy when you have all that extra time at night to heal your fears?

Or will the subconscious suddenly find an association you had been missing? Will a dream reveal that the reason you feared cats was because of a forgotten childhood experience? Perhaps your boss's voice reminds you of someone who hurt you, but it was not in your conscious awareness. When you can understand the origin of fear, you can make sense of your experience. As you learned in the last chapter, that's the left side of the brain turning down the overactive right side of the brain. Then, the boost in gamma waves allows "aha" moments to turn gasps of fear into sighs of relief.

It's also possible that the origin of your fear isn't a forgotten memory from your childhood but perhaps the fear from your ancestors, acquired through epigenetic inheritance. In 2014, neuroscientists at Emory conducted a fascinating study pairing the smell of cherry blossoms with shocks to mice. Then, they bred the mice. When their offspring were exposed to cherry blossoms, they became fearful and anxious—despite the fact that only their parents had learned to associate this pleasant smell with an unpleasant sensation. When researchers tested the next generation—the "grandchildren" of the original mice—this generation also became fearful and anxious when exposed to the smell of cherry blossoms.[6]

If you fear something because your parents or grandparents learned it was scary, is it possible that SVT could help you rewind the tape to early childhood? Perhaps you'll remember a forgotten story your mother told you when you were a little girl or boy.

Would you like the sound of that jet taking off to remind you of your belief that everything in this world makes sense in some grand way? Some part of you knows that already, doesn't it? After all, you now know that your subconscious has been conspiring in your favor. Perhaps you're starting to see that the universe does the same thing.

Maybe your boss's voice is going to remind you of your true grace. At some point, you'll probably be reminded that the people who are hardest to love are the ones who need love the most. In your profession, will you be reminded of why you do what you do? Maybe you'll work a little harder on that side hustle—so it can become your nine-to-five one day. I'm not sure what the ultimate answer will be for you . . . only you and your subconscious know the answer. But it will be so rewarding to find out.

Of course, I'll help you build a bridge to carry this experience into waking life. You'll have an image or a sound that will trigger your brain's inner pharmacy whenever you need a dose of GABA to calm you. Won't that be so nice? You could have a built-in drip for Xanax on your finger . . . and you didn't even know it. (It can be a morphine drip, too. More on that in the pain chapter.)

SVT to Stress Less & Conquer Fears

Activating the subconscious brain is a simple shift from your fight-or-flight mode to your rest-and-digest mode, which makes it an incredible tool to transform stress into serenity. When you have 30 to 40 minutes, read the instructions for step 1 below and then listen to the audio track "SVT to Stress Less & Conquer Fear" (see page 242 for download information). I recommend practicing SVT at the end of the day, so that you are free to remain in a relaxed state of mind or even fall asleep after the practice. Especially for stressing less and conquering your fears, why not let this practice usher into a restful night's sleep?

You'll do step 1 again now as a stand-alone practice as it specifically relates to stress and fear. Then, steps 2 through 7 are done as one seamless practice—as peacefulness washes over you.

- Step 1: Considering the Conscious
- Step 2: Activating the Subconscious
- Step 3: Revising the Past
- Step 4: Enhancing the Present
- Step 5: Creating the Future
- Step 6: Planting Positivity
- Step 7: Building Bridges

Stress and fear vie for your attention every day, sometimes as soon as you sit up in bed or your feet hit the floor. Wouldn't it be so nice to get a jump on those situations? You could use this SVT practice as a preventative tonic for stress in the morning if you allow at least 30 minutes. Or after a particularly stressful day, use it in the evening. Soon, you'll notice how easy and natural remaining calm becomes.

STEP 1: CONSIDERING THE CONSCIOUS

In Chapter 3, you wrote down the three pitfall thought patterns that plague you the most. Now go back to those thought patterns (page 47). As it relates to stress and fear, which one pitfall or negative mantra causes the most anxiety, stress, or fear? Write it down here:

Type of pitfall thought pattern: _____

_____

which, to me, is a thought that sounds something like: _____

_____

Now that your conscious brain knows what it needs to change, allow your powerful subconscious brain to figure out how it will change it.

STEPS 2 THROUGH 7: STRESS LESS AND CONQUER FEAR

I've included this written SVT script for you to come back to when you become advanced so you can practice without the guided audio tracks. It's also a blueprint for practitioners training in SVT. In a comfortable seated or lying posture, listen to audio track "SVT to Stress Less & Conquer Fear" (see page 242 for download information).

I invite you to begin this practice by allowing the eyes to close as you settle in here . . . as the body finds the most comfortable po-

sition to rest. And as you settle here, make any last adjustments if you'd like, resting into this peaceful state of pure serenity . . . I wonder if you can bring your attention to the place in the body where you feel the most relaxed. You already know how to activate the subconscious, which has always been here conspiring in your favor, so let's begin this journey now with some mindfulness. Ever so easily invite yourself to simply notice what's on your mind—right here and right now.

Ever so gently inviting yourself to simply notice what's on your mind—right here and right now. Instead of judging the thoughts, clinging to them, reacting to them, or becoming one with them, you can just gently let them float on by. Isn't it so interesting that when you watch your thoughts in this kind of way, this "thought watching" can start to feel relaxing? You've already begun to transform the thoughts that used to block a sense of calmness into a practice that promotes it. In the future, you'll probably find that this gentle thought watching may become a great place to begin your journey of finding more peace in your everyday life. Wouldn't that be nice? The very thoughts that used to put you into a tailspin can be used to set you free.

*Now pivot your attention to the sense of hearing. Now invite the ears to notice **three sounds** you're hearing right here and right now. That's right. It could be interesting to begin with the loudest sound you can perceive in this moment. Now find a noise that's neither loud nor soft, a medium sound. Now, I wonder what is the quietest sound you can hear . . . can you hear yourself breathing? That's right. Perfect.*

*And now invite the eyes to notice **two colors** you can see on the back of the eyelids. The first being directly in front of you . . . and then, on the next inhale, what color can you see near the crown of the head as you roll the eyes up, up, up?*

On the next exhale, allow the eyes to float down, down, down . . . and then just allowing the eyes to relax as any lingering tightness simply floats away. Yes, that's right. And now I invite *you to really feel **one breath**. Allowing the breath to breathe you. Can you feel the breath rocking you? Can you feel the place where the breath feels the most peaceful? Allow that feel-good or soothing sensation to spread through the brain and body. That's right. Perfect.*

As you tune in to your senses, rooted in this present moment, you will probably find that the judgment, scrutiny, and defenses of the conscious begin to float away. And you are reminded that the subconscious is always looking out for you; it sees your greatest potential today and what possibilities you can look forward to tomorrow. Throughout this healing journey, you may also find that images and memories are more vivid and lifelike when viewed through the lens of the subconscious.

And with that, it's also nice to be reminded that you are the observer of everything that unfolds here, isn't it? Remember, you always have the power to minimize or close a screen. Or, if you'd like, mute the volume . . . all the things you now know how to do. Isn't it nice to know you're in control at all times, here, in this practice? Most people say this enhanced sense of control stays with them even when this formal practice has come to an end.

I invite you to send a message to the subconscious right now that today, you're only going to see, hear, and experience what you're ready to see, hear, and experience. Call upon the subconscious right now, and softly ask it to help you in the way you most need today.

Isn't it so nice to know your subconscious is conspiring in your favor and always knows what you need to heal? It knows what baby step you're ready to take today, and perhaps it knows what step you will take tomorrow. Or perhaps it will take that step for you tonight as you're dreaming. And it will all feel so easy and effortless.

In just a moment, but not quite yet, you'll use the power of your mind's eye to see and feel yourself going down an escalator with

12 floors. See yourself at the top of this escalator. . . . That's right. You can see it, can't you? What color is it? You already have a sense that this journey will be a calming and comfortable one.

See and feel yourself gliding down this escalator now.

12. *Beginning to feel a deep sense of relaxation washing over you. That's right.*

11. *As you feel yourself moving down the escalator, you'll become twice as calm as you were the floor before.*

10. *Simply allow the body to take all the time it needs. Many people notice the breath becoming slower and more relaxed here. I wonder if you may notice your breath moving down into your belly, as it does when the subconscious begins to take over. That's an indication that you're more relaxed. As the breath slows, the mind calms.*

9. *I wonder if you can actually feel a sense of the body moving down . . . so steady and so serene. And as you do, you're becoming cool, calm, and comfortable.*

8. *Perhaps noticing now how this relaxation may help you to let go of any tightness in your body. And as that happens, your mind easily lets go of any remnants of conscious thought or worry. That's right. Good.*

7. *Even more deeply calm now. It's almost as if every floor this escalator glides down helps you to become two or even three times more relaxed and comfortable than you were on the floor before. And when that happens, I wonder if you'll notice how nice this all feels. Perfect.*

6. *Halfway down now. That's right. Letting go a bit more now. Isn't that such a nice feeling? You deserve this rest. After all, you do so much in your everyday life, don't you?*

5. *Almost there now, and you may notice that the mind embodies the same easy "rag doll" quality as you may feel now in the body. Your brain no longer has to do anything. I wonder if you have already begun to feel as though there's something that you were meant to overcome today. Either way, it can be so incredible just to have this time to really rest and relax.*

4. *Feeling yourself glide down to the next floor now, you may notice a wonderful dreamlike state come to you—now or at some point in this journey.*

3. *Almost there now. That's right. You're doing so wonderfully already . . . and you've only just begun.*

2. *Gliding down, next-to-last floor now. Perfect. Feeling twice or maybe even three times as calm, dreamy, or relaxed on this step as you were on the floor before.*

1. *Notice now . . . where in the brain or body do you feel the most relaxed? If you'd like, allow that relaxation to spread over the rest of you, especially to the place you need it most. Just take all the time you'd like here to enjoy this type of experience you're feeling now. That's right. Very good.*

Now that you've felt the body make its way down the escalator, you've probably noticed the brain begin to slow itself down into a state of healing relaxation.

In just a moment, you'll feel the body start to float upward as your consciousness begins to expand and I count up from one to seven. As these two things happen—body floating and consciousness expanding—you may notice an even deeper sense of peace and relaxation.

As the body floats, many people also notice it feels warm, as though you're taking a warm bath or floating in the ocean on a summer day. As you practice this more, you may even find that you lose a sense of time and space. You may even find that—if you'd like—you can create a sense of "leaving" the physical body for this healing time you've given yourself. If it feels comfortable, you may wish to see your consciousness actually leaving the physical body as a momentary "out-of-body" experience. Your consciousness will return effortlessly at the end of this practice . . . or at any time you'd like.

Counting now:

1. *Body float.*

2. *Consciousness moving upward and expanding so that it's now larger than the body.*

3. *Body becoming lighter and warmer.*

4. *Consciousness moving upward and expanding even more so that it fills the room.*

5. *Body becoming almost weightless now.*

6. *Consciousness so elevated and expanded that it's joining with the universe.*

7. *So deep and so relaxed. Perfect.*

Now I invite you to ask your subconscious to help you by visualizing a person or a scene that will help you feel safe, peaceful . . . and calm. Will this be a person, or will it be an energy you take on this healing journey?

If it's a person, you may wish to see him or her next to you. Would you like to see this person taking your hand? It's so nice to know you're not alone, and it's also so comforting to know that you're in control. That's right. If you see a feeling or a kind of energy in your mind's eye, perhaps you can feel yourself taking some part of this and stitching it around the heart or stuffing a bit of it in a pocket. That's right. Perfect.

Now I'd like you to imagine that you see a blank canvas in front of you. Perhaps this blank canvas represents the screen that your subconscious projects your dreams onto—like an outdoor movie screen. In just a moment, but not quite yet, I'm going to have you project an image onto that screen.

Remember that your subconscious is also taking care of you—so it won't show you anything that you're not ready to see. You may use this same script 10 times, and every time, it may show you a little bit more. Isn't that so comforting? That's your subconscious taking care of you . . . your own inner mother to your inner child. This experience is going to help you stress less and find serenity.

You see, today's stressors are often a result of yesterday's memories. Something or someone stresses you out, and you don't know why. Who does he or she remind you of? Why is this getting to you? Is it a particular memory, or is it simply something deeper about who you are . . . something about who you respond to and why? Why is it you are so afraid of this or that—or any type of situation that is scary to you? Your brain probably paired a memory with a feeling of being scared. Oh, that's right. It was your aunt's old cat . . . that's why you're so afraid of cats today.

Or maybe—just maybe—this fear is something that happened to one of your ancestors. After all, you now know that fear can be encoded and inherited. That is, after all, where our instinctual fears come from, isn't it? And if there were a key to access this door to see it, it would be here—through the subconscious. So if you believe that you can see your ancestors' fears, then you could—if you'd like—see even that.

And so I'm going to ask your subconscious now to rewind the tape as far back as you need to go—to the very first time you felt this way. In front of you is that blank canvas. In just a moment, I'm going to count from three down to one . . . and then you'll hear me snap my fingers. . . . When you hear that snap, your subconscious is going to project the root of your stress, anxiety, or fear—the first time you felt this way . . . or at least as much as you're ready to see today. In some cases, the origin may be quite simple. In others, it may be complex. With openness, simply allow your subconscious to find the scene or the images.

Three . . . two . . . one. [snap]

What do you see on your screen?

Do you see the root of your stress, fear, or anxiety, or are you simply reminded of something you already knew about yourself? For most people, simply knowing the root of the fear or stress is already calming in and of itself. Did you have a small—or perhaps even a significant—"aha" moment?

Now, most people experience some side-to-side eye flutter as they relax throughout the SVT practice. As I count backward from three to one, allow your eyes to relax, and the eyes will flutter left and right just a bit more. And this time, play the scene or scenes you found from the beginning to the end . . . and if you get to the end, simply loop it around to begin again. Pressing play and allowing the eyes to flutter now on three . . . two . . . one.

Now inhale on the count of three: one, two, three. Exhale on the count of six: one, two, three, four, five, six. Many people notice tension, but at least one or two places in the body will feel at ease. Now, as I count from one to five, the subconscious brain will spread that ease to the rest of the mind, body, and spirit: one, two, three, four, five. That's right. Perfect.

Now, this time I invite you to review the same scene. But this time, simply notice everything you already did to handle the stress fairly well. As you throw that same scene up onto the blank canvas of your mind's eye, really see all the things you did to help yourself feel safe and secure. Isn't it nice to consider what you're already doing right? In this relaxed and comfortable state, you'll probably also notice how your breath is beginning to migrate down to the belly and become slow and steady, which is a sign that you are in a wonderful state we call "rest-and-digest." Notice; where in your body do you feel the most calm right now? Isn't it so wonderful to know that you're already pairing a state of calm with these images?

So in just a moment, when you press play, you'll do two things. First, see this scene—how you handled the stress fairly well. Second, notice where in your body you feel most calm. Pressing play and inviting the eyes to flutter side to side now on three . . . two . . . one [left-right-left-right audio tones].

Now inhale on the count of three: one, two, three. Exhale on the count of six: one, two, three, four, five, six. Many people notice tension, but at least one or two places in the body feel at ease. Now, as I count from one to five, the subconscious brain will spread that ease to the rest of the mind, body, and spirit: one, two, three, four, five. That's right. Perfect.

And now it's time to imagine that you have access to advanced editing software and wires that only the subconscious can touch. I wonder what the subconscious brain would like to do to that scene. Imagine it's accessing that panel right now and visualizing all these things happening—right here, right now. Are you transforming the cat that looked big and scary into a tiny, happy cartoon character? Or are you turning the volume down on the scene from your past? Would you like to turn those loud sounds that your brain initially encoded as "fear" into sounds that suddenly sound funny? In this moment, how are you reprogramming your brain? Perhaps you'd like to unlearn an association so you will not notice things that cause you stress or fear. Or would you like to tell the brain that the thing that you thought was nasty is actually nice? Either way, it's rather interesting how many things you can change via the subconscious brain. You can use the creativity of your subconscious to do anything you'd like. It knows how best to take care of you. In just a moment, the power of the subconscious brain will start to set you free. And again, notice—in this wonderfully relaxed state—where in your body you feel the most relaxed. That's right. Perfect.

This time, project that movie again. And allow the subconscious to edit the scene in any way it likes. Edit the scene. That canvas is in front of you, and your subconscious is the artist—just like the blank canvas of the dreams you see every night. Again, allow the eyes to flutter side to side as you press play . . . and also edit or delete or mute or whatever you'd like now on three . . . two . . . one [left-right-left-right audio tones].

Now inhale on the count of three: one, two, three. Exhale on the count of six: one, two, three, four, five, six. Many people notice tension, but at least one or two places in the body feel at ease. Now, as I count from one to five, the subconscious brain will spread that ease to the rest of the mind, body, and spirit: one, two, three, four, five. That's right. Perfect.

And now allow the subconscious brain to fast-forward to present day. Isn't it so interesting that the subconscious brain has already begun to set you free? Was it the way it helped you to connect the dots, or was it the way it helped you to see how you're already doing fairly well in managing your life? What was it for you?

Take a moment to notice what feels different now. I don't know if the difference will be a subtle one or a significant one, but you will notice something right now or tomorrow afternoon. Isn't it so interesting that in this moment, you may even be able to find one or two pieces of evidence that you are actually stronger, calmer, and more courageous than you realized?

And in this moment, it's as though you're floating on a cloud. You know—right here and right now, in this calm, cool, confident, courageous, and comfortable state—that you are so much stronger than you realize. The avoidance that you had previously been using to manage your fears or your stress was simply a coping mechanism, wasn't it? Avoidance is only necessary as a way to keep yourself safe when you have no other way to handle your fear . . . but now you know how, don't you? You've changed. You can feel it, can't you? And you've tapped into the strength that allows you to go through it—not around it. And by doing so, you are setting yourself free.

Now, right here and right now . . . as you reflect upon who you are today, I wonder what situation or moment will help you to remember just how strong you are. You see that, don't you? And when you find that memory that reminds you of this strength, then the avoidance and fear you had been using will begin to evaporate. Isn't that incredible? When you remember how capable and brave you are, you don't need your fear anymore, do you? I wonder what memory your subconscious has shown you in this moment that is helping you to access your inherent strength and courage.

Now consider that pitfall thought pattern or negative mantra you wrote down in step 1. I wonder what part of this experience has loosened your belief—has the subconscious transformed that pessimism and its catastrophic, worst-case-scenario thinking into optimism? At this point in the practice, most people find that they already begin to consider the probable more than the possible—and this works wonders when it comes to freeing themselves from fear. Isn't that so nice to know? Perhaps there used to be a mantra. Did you used to walk around the world with one that sounded like, "I'm not okay"? At this point, you are starting to realize that, yes, you are okay . . . and will be even more so in the future. Now imagine a dial of peacefulness. See yourself turning up that dial now. All the way up . . . from five to six to seven. All the way up to 10. That's right. Doesn't that help you to feel so calm? So peaceful?

And now, as you fast-forward the tape with your mind's eye, see yourself in your future. With the confidence of everything that you have already done, see yourself taking a baby step in your life—something that will help you to conquer fear, to become even more free. The power of the subconscious helps you to see this as if it's unfolding right here and right now. And when that's true, it's as if you Jedi-mind-tricked your brain into thinking you've already conquered your fears. If you'd like, you could even supercharge this step with photos or videos— allowing the eyes to float open just a bit during this part of SVT if there's a phobia you're conquering. Make your brain believe it's coming in contact with that cat or anything else it wants to conquer. You know you can now, don't you? Or you can simply allow your subconscious to create the virtual reality of being your calm, confident, courageous self in front of the thing you fear or easily handling the thing that used to cause you stress. That's right. Perfect.

What baby step comes after that? See it now. If it's a matter of stressing less . . . what will you do just a bit differently in the future to stress less? Will your boss's voice remind you of all the patience and grace you already know you have? I wonder, will that yoga class become more of a priority? I wonder if you simply won't notice a former stressor. Have you reprogrammed something and recategorized it as something else, and now it's underneath the umbrella that says "these things are nice"? When you recategorize experiences in that way, it also gives you the opportunity to have positive experiences in the future—so the visualizations you just saw become reality. Also, just give yourself a bit of credit for all the things you do to take care of yourself—like this practice today. And as you do, gently bring your attention to the place in the body where you feel the most relaxation.

And isn't it so nice to know that the subconscious brain will always be looking for opportunities to continue this healing? I wonder if it will continue to show you things you could do differently in your dreams. Many people will have the most pleasant dream after they recategorize formerly nasty objects into nice ones. That's funny. Where did that dream come from?

Will the subconscious show you all the opportunities to create change in your daily life—from yoga to practicing SVT more often to meditation to exercise to more brain-balancing foods? It's so wonderful to realize that you have so much you can change.

In just a moment, I'll have you deepen this relaxation one more time—so that the seeds of positivity will be planted deep in the subconscious. Now deepening this wonderful feeling of being calm and comfortable on three . . . two . . . one. That's right.

Reflect on the fact that you've already done so much today to heal, haven't you? It will be interesting to notice if the changes you feel will be immediate when this practice is over or if you'll notice them next Tuesday afternoon. There will be a time when you will be presented with an image or a voice, and right here and right now, I invite you to call upon your subconscious to pair that image or voice with the most calming part of today's practice. In the future, it will be so interesting to notice how this image or sound will be an instant reminder of this calming feeling. It will be as if it's now a cue for your brain to release its inner pharmacy of relaxing chemicals—your own Xanax, if you will. And I wonder what feeling or strength of yours will also pair with this image or sound or experience? Will it be a reminder of your courage? Or will it be your patience and grace? If your subconscious thinks it's best for you, it may even decide to make whatever you don't need totally unrecognizable, invisible, silent, or forgotten the moment after you see it or hear it hear it. . . . Won't that be interesting? Any comment that prevented a sense of peace and calm will now suddenly become like words in a foreign language . . . so it's as though you'll only be able to hear words of kindness from that person.

If there is something that used to cause fear, but it is something that would be safe to become totally blind or deaf to, you could choose to no longer notice this object . . . or change it. I wonder if this known object will suddenly become a foreign thing that you've never seen or encountered before, like you're on another continent—you're greeting this wonderful, furry creature for the first time. Wouldn't it be so interesting to have a fresh start? Perhaps that sound will become silent, or you may lose that type of hearing . . . keeping your sense of hearing for only all the noises you need to sense to truly keep you safe. Will your brain still hear real smoke alarms? Yes. Will it hear sounds or become sensitive to signals that make your overactive inner smoke detector go off too quickly? No. Won't that be so comforting?

In any case, I know your subconscious has probably already figured out the best way to take care of you. . . . Isn't that so nice to know? You have found something healing here today that will help you. I wonder what that has been here, today, for you and your brain. You have already planted so much in terms of healing calm and comfort. I wonder what day or time it will be when you truly notice that this healing has bloomed.

Now it's time to build a bridge so you can take everything you've gained from this practice into your waking, everyday life. Whenever you need to be reminded of anything and everything you have discovered here, you'll have a way to do so. The first part of building this bridge involves a button.

First, I want you to find the three best things you've gained here. Perhaps they were lessons or insights. I wonder if they were energies or feelings; you could even visualize them as colors if you'd like. Now send the best part of what you've gained down your dominant arm into your dominant hand. Gather and intensify the feeling of calmness or courage into your dominant index finger. That's right. Now rub the tip of that index finger with that thumb. Can you feel that? There. You've just built a button for yourself. In your waking, everyday life, whenever you need a little piece of what you've created here, all you need to do is push that button. All the feelings, lessons, or sense of freedom will come flooding back. If you come into contact with a stressor and need a little extra boost of a stress-relieving brain chemical, all you need to do is press that button. Isn't it so nice to know this button is here for you at any time?

Second, gather any residual stuff you'd like to get rid of—fear, stress, tension, anxiety, or the feeling of being stuck. Now I invite you to visualize that a balloon is tied to your nondominant index finger. Can you feel it? See that balloon being blown up as you fill it with that "hot air" that fuels your stress, fear, and anxiety. Many people may even notice that the finger may even begin to lift a bit here on its own. Isn't that interesting? Just one last moment here. Is there one last ounce of stress or fear you'd like to send into that balloon? That's right.

Now rub that thumb against your nondominant index finger to untie the balloon from your finger. In your mind's eye, see that balloon float far, far away. Can you see it becoming so small? Tiny now? Follow it until it's gone.

Whenever you notice any of this stress, fear, or tension creeping into your waking life, all you need to do is put it into this balloon that's tied to the nondominant index finger. Then, rub your thumb to untie the string . . . and let it all go. In each and every moment, you have the power to set yourself free.

OPTIONAL RE-ALERT

Now see yourself gliding up that escalator. You'll become twice as alert and awake as you move up every floor. You'll return back to your everyday, waking state as your consciousness returns fully to your body. That's right.

1. *Feel yourself becoming alert as you glide up now.*

2. *Becoming more and more awake as you ascend.*

3. *Perhaps giving a wiggle to your fingers and your toes, and as you do, feel more and more alert.*

4. *That's right. More activated as you glide up.*

5. *Twice as energized and awake as you were the floor before.*

6. *Gliding up again.*

7. *Really feel an increased sense of energy, and feel your consciousness return to your body.*

8. *That's right.*

9. *Alert and activated . . . and wiggling those fingers and toes a bit more now.*

10. *Feeling your body ascend.*

11. *Almost there.*

12. *Eyes open. And when they do, you feel completely rejuvenated, rested, and relaxed.*

To ensure you're fully conscious again, look around the room and name aloud 10 items you see, take a walk around the block, listen to some upbeat music, or do 25 jumping jacks.

CHAPTER 9

SVT to Boost Your Mood

It's probably easy to understand how SVT could undo the pairing of something you've learned, like seeing a cat and feeling scared. But mood—that feels more hardwired, right? You're born with a genetically influenced tendency for mood that can't be changed. Or . . . are you? If you listen to all the commercials for antidepressants on American TV (which, by the way, are illegal to advertise on television in every other country except New Zealand), that's what they'll talk you into believing. Those drug companies know a lot about human behavior—and how to coerce your brain into thinking that you are depressed and need their drug. You have low serotonin, and their latest pill is just what you need. And maybe they're right. Depression *does* hurt, doesn't it? Maybe you *do* feel more achy lately. Maybe you *do* need that pill.

Isn't it interesting that the drug commercials talk to you in ways that are similar to the phrases you hear during SVT? Of course, there is one obvious difference. The language, images, and even the happy-sounding name of their new pill du jour (e.g., Brintellix, Viibryd, Cymbalta) taps into the subconscious brain's inherent suggestibility to convince you that you need their latest and greatest "happy" pill because you're not okay. On the other hand, SVT helps you tap into your own inner well of resources and strengths—because you are *more okay* than you give yourself credit for.

So can SVT help boost your mood? Yes, SVT is a powerful tool to help you to become more optimistic while helping to lift your spirits. What starts as a suggestion becomes a scientifically valid boost. When you listen to the SVT audio track for this chapter, it will be like you're putting on a pair of rose-colored glasses. These glasses will help you filter the information your brain receives from the outside world. Your brain determines if you filter data through a half-glass-full or a half-glass-empty lens. I imagine you already have an idea which lens your brain prefers, don't you?

Wherever you may be on that spectrum today, SVT has the power to make you a more of a glass-half-full person tomorrow. Wouldn't it be so nice to be more like that friend who's always looking on the bright side? You know the type, that person who is sunny no matter what. Good news: you have that happy-go-lucky person inside your subconscious brain.

THE SCIENCE OF SVT: MOOD BOOSTING

It's true that your genetics plays some role in your mood "set point." However, your set point for mood is usually nature *and* nurture. Life experiences activate your genetic tendencies. While your genes load the gun, it's your situation, choices, and everyday life that pull the trigger. Thus, genes are expressed (also known as being "turned on") in certain ways.

Consider a pair of identical twins who are both glass-half-full people throughout their childhood. Then, Twin A experiences financial hardship, a tough breakup, and job loss in her early 20s. Twin B does not. Twin A may experience depression because the hardships turned on the gene associated with depression.

Every depressive episode a person experiences increases a person's risk for having future problems with mood. That makes sense, doesn't it? When you're in a bad mood, you're more likely to skip all the activities that are linked with well-being: exercise, eating well, socializing, and even making your bed. And so, a downward spiral is born. The runaway train of a bad mood leads to more bad moods.

Sometimes, feelings are information. They say: you need to make a change in your life. It's time to move to a new city or find a new career. But when you get stuck in patterns of unhealthy behavior, then those feelings are no longer reliable. It's like you start seeing the whole world through glasses that need to be cleaned. You start to feel hopeless. You start to lose hope that you'll ever be able to see the world clearly ever again. This creates a negative feedback loop in the brain, which can lead to even more bad moods.

Twin A may experience mood problems for years and become a glass-half-empty person. She now looks at the world through a "nothing ever works out for me" lens. On the other hand, Twin B stays a glass-half-full person; she continues to wear that lens of "the universe conspires in my favor." The brain looks for evidence that affirms either one of these mantras; this confirmation bias is your tendency to interpret situations in a way that provides evidence for your existing belief system.

Test your confirmation bias right now. Look around the room as you say the word *red* to yourself. Do you see how your eye notices the red in the room even though the colors in the room did not change? That's a simple example, but confirmation bias is what often leads us to jump to conclusions. SVT helps you to change the lens so you can use Twin B's type of confirmation bias: looking for the *what's right*. It's like Lasik for your brain.

Go back to page 48. What's your negative mantra? What evidence does your brain find to support it? The incredible thing is that SVT has the power to help *both* twins. Twin B gets even more optimism, positivity, and a boost in mood. What it can do for Twin A is truly astounding: It can help her become a glass-half-full person again. It can short-circuit that runaway train of bad moods, naysaying self-talk, and unhealthy behaviors. SVT lays the tracks to get your brain back on course, creating a new confirmation bias. It transforms that pitfall thought pattern, reprograms your mantra, and makes your behaviors healthier.

> ### Reminder:
>
> This book contains self-guided SVT as a tool for boosting mood. It is not a substitute for inpatient or intensive outpatient treatment when severe mental illness is present. Remember: SVT can also be used with a provider as part of an integrative treatment plan.

Do you also remember the Jedi mind trick of the subconscious brain from the last chapter: the ability to change top-down processing? Wouldn't it be nice to simply *not notice* the triggers of a bad mood? What if I could change rain-on-my-parade-type comments into gibberish so you could only understand compliments? It would be as though you became totally deaf to people's digs. Perhaps you'd also like me to plant positivity so that when you do feel a bit low, you easily and effortlessly go to that yoga class, eat organic kale, and spend time with people who nourish you. If you'd like, I can even suggest that you'll take better care of yourself as you receive harsh feedback or bad news. That way, after a few moments, a less-than-ideal mood simply moves on . . . so you can see the sunshine again.

BUT WHAT ABOUT DEPRESSION?

You already learned how good old-fashioned, tried-and-true CBT is more effective in treating anxiety, fear, and stress when it is supercharged with the subconscious brain. Good news: this has also been proven in depression. A recent study showed that subconscious-based techniques with CBT helped boost the subjects' mood while helping them feel more hopeful. This study divided 84 subjects diagnosed with depression into two groups. Group one was treated with good old-fashioned CBT. Group two got CBT *with* subconscious brain–harnessing techniques. While both groups improved, group two experienced bigger boosts in mood and hope.[1] This is great news for Twin A because this can help her to interrupt the downward spiral of bad moods . . . and unhealthy choices . . . and a pessimistic outlook. . . .

In and of itself, CBT works fairly well in helping people to boost mood and become more a glass-half-full outlook. I encourage pairing the two practices for treating depression—which, of course, is what you'll do by practicing SVT. Martin Seligman's classic book *Learned Optimism* works by targeting three pitfall thought patterns that affect pessimists and people with mood dips. These tend to be different pitfalls than those for people with anxiety (i.e., paralysis by analysis and polarization). One of the main principles in *Learned Optimism* is to change the pitfall thought patterns through the processes that the conscious brain governs. They are:

1. **Permanence:** Optimists believe that negative events are *temporary*, while good things happen for permanent reasons. Pessimists believe the opposite: that gray skies are here to stay and that rainbows are fleeting.

2. **Pervasiveness:** Optimists don't let a bad experience affect all areas of their lives. Optimists keep negative life experiences specific. Pessimists do the opposite: they make negative experiences global. Don't let one piece of dirt muddy the entire pond.

3. **Personalization:** Optimists blame bad events on causes that have nothing to do with them and give themselves credit when good things happen. Pessimists do the opposite: they blame themselves for things that go wrong and don't take personal credit for things that go right.

Changing these pitfall thought patterns via the conscious brain does indeed work. Target the *thought*, and then make a conscious choice to change your *experience*—which changes the thought *and* the way you feel. That's the essence of CBT, and I use these strategies with my patients all the time.

Any thought that doesn't lift you up will effortlessly begin to dissipate like fog rolling off a meadow in the early morning.

But wouldn't it be nice if you could make those changes even more deep rooted? That's what SVT can help you to do—by harnessing the conscious brain *and* the power of the subconscious. Wouldn't it be so nice to suddenly become an optimist? Would you like to be reminded that any gray sky will soon give way to sunshine? Or perhaps you need some positivity planted so that you'll effortlessly take part in activities that make you happy—even when something didn't go your way. I wonder if you'd like to be reminded of how *capable* and *confident* you are . . . so that any thought that doesn't lift you up will effortlessly begin to dissipate like fog rolling off a meadow in the early morning.

A TREMENDOUS TRIO

Let's take a brief look at how the conscious and subconscious brain work in lifting your mood. CBT works by pointing out what you're doing "wrong," your "errors" in thinking. Then, it helps you talk back to the naysaying tapes playing in your head. That's a really good thing because that itty bitty shitty committee now has someone standing up to it. Another proven strategy I use frequently is mindfulness. The evidence-based protocol of Mindfulness-Based Cognitive Therapy (MBCT) treats depression by shifting the person to a place of open-minded nonjudgment. Instead of talking back to the negative thoughts, mindfulness helps you to simply let them float by. I am a huge fan of mindfulness meditation and MBCT.

Interestingly, those two tools also use different brain waves to create change. CBT is using conscious thought and thus beta and alpha brain waves. Mindfulness helps to consciously slow the brain down through meditation, creating change mostly with alpha brain waves. SVT goes even deeper, slowing down the brain into a theta-dominant state, where deep-rooted change is uniquely possible.

As you now know, SVT contains elements of both CBT and mindfulness. This is not a polarized either/or way of looking at which one works. It's a way to integrate all these evidence-based tools. The first step also involves a brief flyby of what you're doing "wrong." But the subconscious brain likes positives and "rights" rather than wrongs. Isn't it nice to focus most of your energy on turning up the positive—without so much focus on the negative?

Instead of talking back to those negative tapes that play in your head or learning how to let them float by, what if you could prevent those old memories from playing in the first place? As you already know, the subconscious's theta brain waves allow you access to the edit, delete, and mute buttons on your memories. It's like taking a boring movie, muting it, and then imagining your funniest self narrating the scene. It totally changes the tone. Even better, you could record a new, optimistic default tape to play in your brain.

Where do negative and naysaying memories come from? Sometimes, it's your father's voice or the voice of the bully on the playground. Other times, that tape may have nothing to do with your past. It may be the result of pure biology. Sometimes, a neurotransmitter, such as glutamate, dopamine, serotonin, or GABA—or even a mix of the chemicals listed above—is too low. But, wait, could it be your diet? After all, B vitamins and probiotics help to manufacture all those feel-good chemical messengers. Would exercising more help, and would you like it to feel natural and easy? Research has proven exercise to be even more powerful than prescription antidepressants. One study of people diagnosed with major depression divided them into three groups: one exercised, one took the prescription antidepressant Zoloft, and a third did both. After four months, all three groups did roughly the same, with the combination group doing the best by a hair. But after 10 months, the difference was clear: only 8 percent of the exercisers noticed their depression return. The groups taking the drug didn't fare nearly as well: 31 percent of the combination group and 38 percent of the Zoloft-only group had continued mood problems.[2] If SVT can help you to make exercise effortless and easy, then it stands to reason that it is even more potent than Zoloft in helping to boost mood.

To use SVT as a part of a holistic and integrative strategy, I recommend testing for neurotransmitter deficiencies and lifestyle changes. If you need more B vitamins to boost serotonin, then SVT can help you eat more healthy foods that are rich in brain-healthy nutrients. That's why SVT is so powerful in helping people create effortless change. You can learn more about testing for neurotransmitter deficiencies and other integrative strategies I recommend at my website, drmikedow.com.

SVT FOR BOOSTING MOOD

Circumstances and relationships change every day, and they can impact your mood. So whether you're dealing with the occasional blues or depression, SVT for boosting mood is worth making a regular practice. Especially if your depression is deep seated, use this SVT in conjunction with visits to a qualified health care professional. The power pair will help undo long-term negativity and pitfall thought patterns.

This time, the seven steps of SVT will help boost your mood. You'll do step 1 again now as a stand-alone practice as it specifically relates to dips in mood. Then, steps 2 through 7 will be one seamless practice that allows a composed sense of contentment to wash over you.

- Step 1: Considering the Conscious
- Step 2: Activating the Subconscious
- Step 3: Revising the Past
- Step 4: Enhancing the Present
- Step 5: Creating the Future
- Step 6: Planting Positivity
- Step 7: Building Bridges

STEP 1: CONSIDERING THE CONSCIOUS

Consider those three pitfall thought patterns you wrote down on page 47. As it relates to dips in mood, is there one pitfall thought pattern in particular that is linked to these dips? Is it a thought pattern that prevents you from making it to that yoga class or eating yams? Perhaps when you review the thought patterns on page 44, you'll recognize a new pitfall that is tied to your dips in mood. As you know, permanence, pervasiveness, and personalization are all happiness blockers.

Write this pitfall thought pattern down here:

Type of pitfall thought pattern: _____

which, to me, is a thought that sounds something like: _____

Now that your conscious brain knows what it needs to change, allow your powerful subconscious brain to figure out how it will change it.

STEPS 2 THROUGH 7 OF SVT FOR BOOSTING MOOD

In a comfortable seated or lying posture, listen to the audio track "SVT for Boosting Mood" (see page 242 for download information) to boost your mood and battle depression.

I invite you now to begin this practice by allowing the eyes to close as you settle in here . . . as the body finds the most pleasant position in which to relax and recharge. And as you settle here, make any last adjustments if you'd like, resting into this nice, satisfying state. . . . I wonder if you can bring your attention to the place in the body where you feel the most comfortable, the most calm. You already know how to activate the subconscious, which has always been here, conspiring in your favor, so I invite you to begin this journey simply with some mindfulness. Ever so easily invite yourself to simply notice what's on your mind— right here and right now.

You already know how to activate the subconscious brain . . . and in just a moment, we'll walk through this process again.

If you'd like, you could picture each one of your thoughts or feelings as clouds that you see floating above you. And isn't it so nice just to notice each cloud . . . and then allow that cloud to float on by? Greet each cloud with a gentle "I see you." Isn't it nice that you don't have to do anything with that cloud? You can just notice it. You can just watch it. After all, there's nothing to bother you and nothing to do in this relaxed state. I wonder when you'll notice that next cloud floating toward you. Moment by moment. Cloud by cloud.

Many people say this helps them to develop a new relationship to their thoughts and feelings over time . . . which helps them to feel a bit better. For others, it helps them to feel a lot better. It doesn't really matter exactly how much better you'll feel . . . there's no need to quantify it. After all, this new space is actually a space where all judgment—including the conscious brain's way of appraising thoughts or feelings—floats away like these clouds. Isn't that so nice? If any of this feels relaxing or recharging for you, then your subconscious brain can picture thoughts and feelings as clouds whenever you'd like.

Perhaps you also realize that clouds are actually a lot like thoughts and feelings, aren't they? Like clouds, thoughts and feelings come and go. And just as your brain is always remembering and forgetting at any moment—so it can forget this in order to remember that—the brain also has to make room for new experiences, and new thoughts, and new feelings. . . . It's thinking and feeling this way now as it experiences this. In a moment, it will be thinking and feeling another way when it experiences that.

I'm not sure exactly what your clouds will look like at this moment, but what I do know is that the sky never looks exactly the same. That's the beauty of this ever-changing sky and all these clouds. Do you see a lot of clouds in your sky at this moment . . . or just a few? I wonder if you're able to notice any dark clouds you see with the same type of openness as you do the white, fluffy ones. I wonder what your sky looks like right here and right now. Isn't it nice to remember that when you see a dark, ominous, or stormy cloud, it also means that there will soon be a rainbow . . . or sunshine . . . or clear skies up ahead? After all, that's what happens after storms, isn't it? In this moment, there's nothing to do but simply watch and notice your clouds . . . with nothing to bother you . . . and nothing to do.

*Now pivot your attention to the sense of hearing. And invite the ears to sense **three sounds** you're hearing right here and right now. That's right. It could be interesting to begin with the loudest sound you can perceive in this moment. And now find a noise that's neither loud nor soft, a medium sound. Now, I wonder what's the quietest sound you can hear. . . . Can you hear your breath? That's right. Perfect.*

*And now invite the eyes to notice **two colors** you can see on the back of the eyelids. The first being directly in front of you . . . and then, on the next inhale, what color can you see near the crown of the head as you roll the eyes up, up, up?*

On the next exhale, allow the eyes to float down, down, down . . . allowing any lingering tightness to just float away as you allow the eyes to just relax. Yes, that's right. And now I invite *you to really feel **one breath**. Allowing the breath to breathe you. Where does the breath feel the most pleasant? Where does it feel the warmest? Can you feel the nostrils being warmed by two degrees? Or the lungs contracting by two millimeters? That's right. That's right. Perfect. Just allowing any feel-good sensation you notice to spread through you. That's right . . .*

I invite you to call upon the subconscious and ask it to help you make a change in the way you need it most today. Would you like to have a rosier attitude in the way you see things, or does the subconscious know that it'd be most helpful for you to create positive changes in the way you live your daily life—or would you like it to do both? Isn't it nice that by giving this time to yourself, it's a way of you saying, "I deserve this . . . I'm worthy," which, of course, is something your subconscious already knows.

*In just a moment, but not quite yet, I'll invite you to use the power of your mind's eye to see and feel yourself descend **12 floors** in an elevator. Can you see it in front of you? That's right. What kind of elevator is it? Is it an old one or a modern one? Or if you'd like, you can transform your "elevator" into a floating cloud that you'll step onto . . . and perhaps that cloud is going to gently help you to float down to an even deeper state of pleasant relaxation. Perhaps you'll even find a sense of purpose on this healing journey.*

See and feel yourself boarding that elevator now. Can you see yourself pressing the number one?

12. Beginning to feel a pleasant sense of relaxation washing over you. That's right.

11. As you feel yourself descending, you'll become twice as calm as you were on the floor before.

10. Simply allow the body to take all the time it needs. Perfect.

9. I wonder if you can actually feel a sense of the body floating down.

8. *Perhaps noticing now how this relaxation may help you to let go of any tightness in your body. That's right.*

7. *It's almost as if every floor you descend can help you to become two or even three times more relaxed and comfortable as you were on the floor before. Perfect.*

6. *Halfway down now. That's right. Letting go a bit more now. Isn't that such a nice feeling?*

5. *Almost there now, and you may notice that the mind embodies the same easy "rag doll" quality as you may feel now in the body.*

4. *Feeling yourself move to the next floor down, you may notice a pleasant dreamlike state come to you—now or at some point in this journey.*

3. *Almost there now. That's right. You're doing so wonderfully already . . . and you've only just begun.*

2. *Next-to-last floor. Perfect. Feeling twice or maybe even three times as calm as on the floor before.*

1. *Notice now . . . where in your body do you feel the most relaxed? If you'd like, allow that relaxation to spread over the rest of you, especially to the place you need it most. Just take all the time you'd like here to enjoy this type of experience you're feeling now. That's right. That's fine.*

Now that you've felt the body make its way down these floors, you've probably noticed the brain begin to slow itself down into a state of healing relaxation.

In just a moment, you'll feel the body start to float upward as your consciousness begins to expand and I count up from one to seven. As these two things happen—body floating and consciousness expanding—you may notice an even deeper sense of peace and relaxation.

As the body floats, many people also notice it feels warm, as though you're taking a pleasant, warm bath or floating in the ocean on a summer day. As you practice this more, you may even find that you lose a sense of time and space. You may even find that—if you'd like—you can create a sense of "leaving" the physical body for this healing time you've given yourself. If it feels comfortable, you may wish to see your consciousness actually leaving the physical body as a momentary "out-of-body" experience. Your consciousness will return easily by the end of this practice or at any time you'd like.

Counting now:

1. Body float.

2. Consciousness moving upward and expanding so that it's now larger than the body.

3. Body becoming lighter and warmer.

4. Consciousness moving upward and expanding even more so that it fills the room.

5. Body becoming almost weightless now.

6. Consciousness so elevated and expanded that it's joining with the universe.

7. So deep and so relaxed. Perfect.

Now I invite you to ask your subconscious to help you. Accessing a memory and floating back to a time you felt truly content, truly satisfied. I don't know if your sense of contentment will feel like a quiet peace or if it will be more like joy . . . your subconscious already knows the kind of energy you need most right now. And I wonder if you can see and taste and smell this all—as if it's happening right now. Immerse yourself in this pleasant memory. I wonder: Is there someone there with you? Does some part of you know that you're inherently worthy and good enough in this moment? Does this person help remind you of this . . . or have you tapped into the forgotten belief within yourself?

I don't know exactly what kind of memory or emotion you'll feel right now . . . and it really doesn't matter. What matters is that you remember that you do have the ability to feel content—to feel joy, to feel pleasure—don't you? If you'd like, you can take a piece of this energy or emotion with you through your journey. See and feel yourself putting it in your pocket, or if it's a person who lifts you up, imagine you're putting a locket with that person's photo and words around your neck. Or if you'd like, I invite you to just allow this feeling to wash over every cell in your body. That's right. Perfect. You're doing so wonderfully already.

In just a moment, but not quite yet, I'll ask your subconscious to find the origin of any naysaying voice inside your head. These are those negative tapes that prevent you from reaching your true potential . . . that block you from your happiest, healthiest, and highest self. Now allow your subconscious to float back—like a cloud meandering across the sky of time. One day, one week, one month, one year, and then another year . . . to go back to the first time you felt this way. For some people, the negative tapes that play inside their heads are someone else's voice. Who's telling you you're not good enough? For others, it's going to be a feeling, a time they remember feeling this way. Do you remember the first time you felt really blue . . . perhaps feeling a bit bluer than or different from other people? And as you float back, you'll remember that your subconscious is here to take care of you. And take comfort in knowing that if the memory feels too intense, you can simply float back away from it a bit—like a cloud floating a few feet away from a screen. Now that you have discovered some of the origin of this negative tape inside your head, we'll ask the subconscious to help us change it . . . in just a few moments.

In just a moment, but not quite yet, I'll ask you to play the scene or scenes you found from the start to the finish. Only this time, I'd like you to imagine you're reviewing the scene through rose-colored glasses . . . and I wonder how this will change the tapes inside your head. And as you turn down, delete, or mute any voice that's not serving you, the volume of your own positive self-talk will get turned up. As the tape that plays inside your head becomes more cool, confident, and courageous, I wonder what else will change in the scene. Will you speak up more for yourself . . . and say something different to someone in this scene? Would the wiser version of yourself like to say something to this younger person? Will you become deaf to the voice that doesn't serve you as the voice that lifts you up grows louder? Will you reframe what's happening in a way that is calmer, more proactive? I wonder what you'll do differently this time.

Of course, everyone experiences less-than-ideal situations that we can't entirely control. . . . What you can control is how you handle them . . . and how you talk to yourself. So if you can change the tape inside your head, then you have actually just empowered yourself to face any situation—isn't that wonderful? And as you no longer take people or experiences so personally, they float on by . . . like a cloud.

Let's change that tape right now . . . pressing play on this new, rosier version of the scene as you change the way you talk to yourself . . . and inviting the eyes to flutter side to side a bit more now on three . . . two . . . one . . . [left-right-left-right audio tones].

Now inhale on the count of three: one, two, three. Exhale on the count of six: one, two, three, four, five, six. I wonder if there is a new tape you found in that scene. For most people, the new tape is some version of "I'm good enough" or "I can do it." As I count from one to five, perhaps you could allow this new optimism to wash over every cell in your brain, your body, and your spirit. As you do so, can you feel this new optimism being reprogrammed? Turn that dial up now: one, two, three, four, five. That's right. That's right. Perfect.

Now, in just a moment, but not quite yet, I'll invite you to see that same scene or scenes one more time. When you see the scene this time, I invite you to see how the new, optimistic tape that plays inside your head changes what you would have done. . . see it all unfold in this edited scene. You see, once you change the tape, you're changing the way you feel, and when you change the way you feel, you change the way you act. And isn't it interesting that this new way of being in the world has a snowball effect? After all, people who make choices from a place of confidence tend to create more abundance. Does this new tape of "I'm good enough" allow you to stay confident . . . and not react to the bullies in the scene? Or perhaps a feeling of "I can do this" allows you to keep taking care of yourself—even when you didn't get the support you deserved from others. Isn't it so nice to know that there are so many ways you can take care of yourself? And, of course, this abundance turns into more positive thoughts . . . and those positive thoughts turn into positive feelings—more pleasure, more contentment, more joy, and so on. Isn't it wonderful that you've already begun to create profound change . . . simply by editing the tape inside your head?

So I invite you to press play on that same scene in just a moment. And I wonder how this new, positive tape inside your head changes the way you act . . . in this scene and any life scenes that follow. Allowing the eyes to flutter side to side now as you press play . . . seeing how positive self-talk creates positive action in three . . . two . . . one . . . [left-right-left-right audio tones].

That's right. Perfect. Now inhale on the count of three: one, two, three. Exhale on the count of six: one, two, three, four, five, six. Just notice the place in your body where you feel the most pleasant or energized. Where can you really feel this new tape making a difference in how much better you feel? Take that feeling and turn it up and spread it across your body now as I count from one to five: one, two, three, four, five. That's right. Perfect.

And now I invite the subconscious brain to help you float forward to today. I invite you to see another scene now. It's you in your present life. I wonder if the rose-colored glasses helped you to change something or if you simply gained more understanding of the origin of that old voice you've let go. Of course, the new tape you programmed into your past self is still here with your present self. And so I'd like you to see all the ways this new, positive tape helps you to feel better . . . and do things differently. Yes. That's right . . .

See all the ways the new, more optimistic you will change your present day. I wonder if you begin to notice that any comment that would drag down the old you will sound like gibberish. It's almost as if the subconscious knows exactly how to ignore comments that don't serve your highest self. It also starts to become acutely aware of the comments that will help lift your mood. Wouldn't it be wonderful if these were the only comments you remember—so that positivity and optimism sticks to you like Super Glue . . . while cut-downs simply pass by like a floating cloud? Perhaps you'll be reminded that anyone who is unkind is simply in need of love . . . and from now on, comments or situations that used to drag you down will now become a reminder of your patience and grace. Won't that be so incredible? It will be interesting to see how any less-than-sunny situation now becomes a trigger for all the healing activities you already know how to do. Perhaps you'll go to yoga more or eat more vegetables or volunteer to serve others—whatever that healthy activity is for you. I don't know exactly what you'll do, but your subconscious knows exactly what will help to boost your mood. I wonder when you'll notice that you're doing that activity more.

Now I invite you to really imagine something else. In your mind's eye, imagine that you see three dials in front of you. The first dial is labeled Hope. The second: Optimism. The third: Confidence. Each dial is labeled 1 to 10. Just notice where each of your dials is right now. Isn't that interesting that your sub-

conscious can actually see where those dials are right now? Has the work you've already done turned your dials up a bit already?

And wouldn't it be nice to turn those dials up even more? Isn't it exciting to know that you have the power to turn up these dials . . . and that the subconscious has access to these dials? Some people turn them all the way up to 10; others will just turn them up a notch or two for right now. As you turn up these dials, I wonder what will change for you.

As you turn up that dial for hope, perhaps you'll be struck by the "aha" moment—that dark clouds soon give way to sunny skies. Will this help you know that good things happen for permanent reasons and that negative events float away so easily . . . like clouds in the sky? As you turn up the optimism dial, does it become easier to continue to do things that involve taking care of yourself—even on days when something doesn't go your way—so that your pond of happiness remains mostly clear . . . even when there is a drop of mud? And as the self-worth dial is turned up, I wonder if you will begin to take credit for all the things you do right . . . as events that don't go your way just float on by. You can turn all these dials up as much as you'd like, from a 3 to a 4 . . . and then a 4 to a 6 . . . and then a 6 to an 8 . . . or, if you're ready, all the way up to a 10. See yourself turning up these dials now, and as you do, see the changes—in the way that you talk to yourself, in the way that you feel, and in the way that you act—in your everyday life. That's right. Perfect.

And now that you've turned up these dials, you'll begin to notice that the way you treat yourself begins to change. I wonder how different you'll appear—at dinner parties and at work. Can you even hear more confidence in your voice? Or will people notice that you just seem happier—and is that because you are smiling a bit more or because they can really sense that you are happier? I'm not sure how the changes you already made are going to show up in your daily life, but I do know that the changes you made will show up at some point. For some people, the change is immediate. For others, there will be an experience that occurs in your life—maybe next Wednesday afternoon at 3 P.M. And you'll notice that you're reacting in a much better way. Isn't that interesting?

Now, in your mind's eye . . . just float forward to your future. Can you see how this new tape is helping you create abundance? I wonder how it's helping you reach all those goals. As you see your rosier future, I also invite you now to vividly see the microtasks you'll need to do to get there. You see, changing the tape is just the beginning . . . because that new tape will help you to create momentum and action each and every day. Isn't that exciting? Do you see yourself waking up earlier and taking some time to care for yourself? See this all unfolding . . . right here and right now. Or perhaps you see yourself taking the initiative to plan more social events with friends. You can see it, can't you? I wonder if your subconscious brain is helping you to see yourself exercising . . . and enjoying it . . . and doing it so effortlessly. Your subconscious and your truest self know what activity or changes are right for you.

In this moment, your subconscious brain is breaking down larger goals—and it's showing you all the baby steps you will take each and every day. As you already know, the biggest building is built brick by brick. So as you see yourself in your future now, see every brick. Every morning. Every day. Every year. Isn't it interesting that as you break your goals into these small bricks, it will all start to feel so achievable? Isn't it so nice to know that now that you've seen it unfold, you've used a Jedi mind trick to convince the brain that it can happen . . . because you've already seen it happening? And the brain's bias to confirm what it knows to be true will change the way you see things. I wonder when you'll start to look for and find the evidence that you have the capability and the courage to create anything you see here. That's right. Perfect.

In just a moment, I'll have you deepen this state one more time—so that we can plant the seeds of positivity deep in the subconscious. Now deepening this wonderful feeling of being confident and comfortable on three . . . two . . . one. . . . That's right. I wonder if you'll notice how much you've already done here. Isn't that so nice to just feel—and give yourself credit for? Or is it more exciting that your brain is going to only notice evidence of you being good enough . . . or capable enough? Look at how that tape has already changed. When you return to your everyday life, you'll notice that this new tape has stuck. I don't know if you'll see it right away or in a few days, but there will be something that helps you realize that you're more optimistic or more open. It may even feel as though your lens has changed completely . . . as if you're now viewing the world through these new, rose-colored glasses you put on today. Would you like to keep them on? It will be interesting to see how much more quickly you will bounce back from a cloudy moment. Most people will find some evidence as soon as this practice comes to an end that something deep has become. For others, they'll notice it gradually over the course of days or weeks. I wonder how this change will affect you. And when you notice that, you'll realize that the seeds of change have been planted—because you've planted them—and are beginning to bloom.

And now it's time to build a bridge—so you can take everything you've gained from this practice into your waking, everyday life. Whenever you need to be reminded of anything and everything you have discovered here, you'll have a way to do so. The first part of building this bridge involves a button.

First, I want you to find the three best things you've gained here. Perhaps they were lessons, "aha" moments, or insights. I wonder if they were energies or feelings of self-worth—you could even visualize them as colors if you'd like. Now send the best part of what you've gained down your dominant arm into your dominant hand. Gather and intensify the feeling of calmness or courage in your dominant index finger. That's right. Now rub the tip of that index finger with that thumb. Can you feel that? There. You've just built a button for yourself. In your *waking, everyday life, whenever you need a little piece of what you've created here . . . all you need to do is push that button. All the feelings, lessons, or freedom will come flooding back. If you come into contact with something that is trying to pull you down, all you need to do is press that button. That button will release a little hit of exciting dopamine or calm and confident serotonin. After all, your brain has an inner pharmacy of feel-good chemicals. Isn't it so nice to know this button is here . . . to give you mood-boosting chemicals or a reminder of your inherent strength whenever you'd like?*

Second, gather any residual stuff you'd like to get rid of, any leftover gray feelings or taking things personally or pessimism. Now I invite you to visualize that a balloon is tied to your nondominant index finger. Can you feel it? See that balloon being blown up as you fill it with that "hot air" that fueled any previous dips in mood. Many people notice that the finger may even begin to lift a bit here on its own. Isn't that interesting? Just one last moment here; see if there's one last ounce of sadness or depression or fear you'd like to send into that balloon. That's right. And now rub that thumb against your nondominant index finger—which will untie the balloon from the finger. In your mind's eye, see that balloon float far, far away . . . perhaps you'll even feel that finger floating back down. Can you see the balloon becoming so small? Tiny now? Follow it until it's gone. And in the future, whenever you need to free yourself from negativity, all you need to do is put it into this balloon that's tied to the nondominant index finger. Then, rub your thumb to untie the string . . . and let it all go. In each and every moment, you have the power to set yourself free.

OPTIONAL RE-ALERT

Now see yourself boarding that elevator or that cloud that will take you back up to your life. You'll become twice as alert and awake and return back to your everyday, waking state. You'll feel your consciousness returning to your body. That's right.

1. *Feel yourself becoming alert now.*

2. *As you ascend, become more awake . . . and even excited for everything in store for you and your future. Feeling your consciousness returning to your body.*

3. *Perhaps giving a wiggle to your fingers and your toes and, as you do, feeling more and more awake*

4. *That's right. Up and activated.*

5. *Twice as energized and alert as you were on the floor before.*

6. *Another floor up and feeling so rejuvenated.*

7. *Really feeling all the energy return to your mind and body.*

8. *That's right. So present and so alive.*

9. *Alert and activated . . . wiggling those fingers and toes a bit more now.*

10. *Feeling your body ascend.*

11. *Almost there.*

12. *Eyes open. And when they do, feel excited for this life that is yours to create.*

To ensure you're fully conscious again, look around the room and name aloud 10 items you see, take a walk around the block, listen to some upbeat music, or do 25 jumping jacks.

CHAPTER 10

SVT for Habits and Healthier Living

Perhaps you've heard of people who have used their subconscious brains to go from a pack a day to smoke-free freedom. Case in point: A recent study randomly assigned smokers to one of two groups—eight sessions of hypnosis or no treatment. Six months later, 40 percent of the people who received hypnosis were smoke-free versus 0 percent in the no-treatment group.[1] Would you be surprised to discover that you, too, can tap into the power of your subconscious brain to liberate you from all sorts of habits or create new ones? Whether your vice is a daily pack of Marlboros or a nightly pint of mint chocolate chip, SVT can help you to become smoke-free, sober, or slender. Or perhaps you want healthy habits, but you're struggling to stick with them. Want to be consistent with exercise or your brain-healthy omega-3s? Why not let your subconscious brain do the work for you?

If we look at how habits form in the first place, you'll recognize how both conscious and subconscious parts of your brain are involved. First, some kind of benefit consciously motivates you to make a change or create a discipline: healthier gums by flossing, clear skin by proper hydration, or weight loss by diet and fitness. If you consistently repeat the new practice long enough, usually about four weeks, the repetition lays down new tracks in your brain. So what started as a conscious effort then becomes a subconscious effort, happening on autopilot.

The same mechanisms are at work with unhealthy habits. The two most common root causes are stress management and sensation seeking. Nail biting is an example of a stress management habit. Other examples include hair pulling, scab picking, and pen chewing. Consider a woman who began biting her nails during her divorce. She bites her nails in a desperate attempt to manage her stress and anxiety. The stress may pass, but the repetition of biting her nails becomes habitual. Now, at the first hint of anxiety or stress, she starts nibbling at her fingers. She could be channeling that anxious energy at kickboxing class or by knitting some new outfit for her grandkid.

On the other hand, someone with problematic habits such as gambling, drugs, and sex are sensation seeking. And often their brains process dopamine differently than sensation-avoiding brains. So the thrill someone gets from an occasional jackpot helps him feel normal as his dopamine level spikes and he feels better—for a minute or two. Then, he puts all his winnings—and then some—back in the slot machine. Soon, he's gambled away his rent money. The irony is that, in the long run, the gambling habit is actually depleting his dopamine level, and his brain will develop a tolerance, meaning he'll need more and more dopamine to feel normal.

Unhealthy habits are simply a way for people to get something their brains need. In both these types of habit-bound people, a downward spiral is born. They know they should stop, and they want to stop, but they can't. They've repeated the behavior so often that it's now embedded into their brains. Both are trading short-term comfort for long-term consequences. Any time they try to stop, withdrawal makes them feel worse. They're trapped.

Since the conscious brain tends to analyze unhealthy habits in mathematical ways, it correlates with the pitfall thought pattern of paralysis by analysis, the one that creates worry and increases stress hormones. Then, when you go back to that habit in an effort to feel better . . . you then consciously berate yourself the moment the activity is over. You think, *Why did I do that? What if I'm never able to quit?*

As you know, the subconscious brain works in an entirely different way. SVT can enhance the present as you realize how much in your life is *right*—not *wrong*. It doesn't worry "what if . . ." or dwell on the past. It wonders what opportunities you will create for yourself in the future. Instead of chewing your mangled pen cap as you ruminate on how long you've been trapped in this dead-end job, your subconscious brain helps you visualize the magic you'll create in your new career and see all the steps you'll need to get there. Your fingers aren't twisting that pen with tension. They're typing your application for that writing program.

Seeing the future is vital for anyone cultivating healthier habits. Why? We all need to be reminded that any short-term discomfort we may experience (which, by the way, the subconscious can help you with as well—see Chapter 11 on pain) is a trade-off for long-term health and happiness. Use the power of guided visualization supercharged with the subconscious, and it will feel as though this future is actually unfolding here and now.

Build Your Success

Want to focus more clearly and effectively on your goals? Need help achieving success at work or at home? Turn to the Appendix (page 231) for an SVT practice that will make you more successful in business.

GETTING CONSCIOUS

Before we create a new future of healthy habits, we need to figure out where any deficiencies came from. Some people don't process certain B vitamins in the right way. And B vitamins are needed as "activators" to make neurotransmitters. They make the neurotransmitter serotonin, which helps with stress. And they help make dopamine, which can help make you feel excited. You can learn more about testing for vitamin and neurotransmitter deficiencies on my website (drmikedow.com). It's part of a holistic model of treatment that SVT can support.

But addressing deficiencies is just part of the solution. You see, one tried-and-true strategy for releasing a habit is to consciously remove triggers. This could mean deleting a toxic friend's number from a phone, not keeping cookies in the house, or avoiding sitting down empty-handed in front of the TV—if that means you'll start biting your nails or lighting a cigarette. I've used these helpful strategies with thousands of patients in my private practice. But would you like to take that strategy one step further? Instead of needing to make a conscious effort to avoid certain people, situations, and objects, what if the subconscious could make them vanish completely?

To do that, we need to rewire the brain. SVT allows you to become a master electrician in your brain to gain access to circuits that feed bad habits. Short-circuit connections that aren't serving you, replace burnt-out fuses, and construct a new network that helps you create a happy and healthy life.

Since the subconscious has the ability to tinker with your brain's top-down processing, it's as if you're converting your wiring from an American system to a European one—so your "plugs" don't fit in the "sockets" anymore. As you already know, top-down processing is shaped by what you experience. Through this experiential framework, your brain filters all the bottom-up information coming in from the outside world. Top-down processing can simply discard information that doesn't fit. This can be applied to habits as you Jedi-mind-trick your brain into believing it doesn't know what that striped, rectangular, red-and-white box at the convenience store is, let alone how it tastes. That food that's sabotaging your best efforts for a healthy life morphs into a foreign object.

If eating cookies has become your go-to way of dealing with your stressful job, would you like to become nose-blind to the smell of that bakery next to your office? If daily pot smoking is making your brain feel foggy, what if you no longer recognized that dank smell as you walked by your neighbor's apartment? That'd be nice, wouldn't it? I wonder if, over time, using SVT could save your life. After all, less sugar and fewer carbs means lower likelihood of strokes and cardiovascular problems.

Habit-kicking proof

If you're trying to kick a lifetime habit of smoking or fix that deep rooted desire to devour Häagen Dazs daily, it's unlikely that going to just one session of hypnosis is going to cure you by itself. Research has shown the most effective way to help someone kick a habit is to combine effective tools. That's why SVT includes CBT-based tools and plants suggestions into your subconscious that you keep going to those helpful 12-step meetings. And you may even find them enjoyable again as your subconscious brain helps you keep an eye out for all the ways you can be of service to others in the group, possibly building a life filled with spiritual friendships. Perhaps, it would be nice to feel a great white light of spirituality growing within you.

One study split 286 current smokers into two groups. Both groups got two months' worth of nicotine patches. The first group received CBT, and the second group received hypnosis. While both types of combination therapy were effective, more subjects in the nicotine replacement plus hypnosis group than those in the nicotine replacement plus CBT reported being smoke-free six months later. This was also true after another six months had passed.[2]

SVT begins with CBT and has elements of hypnosis, guided imagery, and suggestions that will supercharge any type of replacement therapy that works for you—whether it's inserting half-marathons into your life as you take Marlboros out, or adding Zumba classes in place of Netflix binges. Thus, SVT takes advantage of all the proven strategies instead of trying just one to make a major change in your life.

Is your habit one that tends to be found in your fridge or accessed by fast food drive-thru windows? When it comes to weight loss, enhancing CBT with the subconscious brain doubles the results. A meta-analysis of studies compared the number of pounds subjects lost with just CBT against pounds lost by subjects who used CBT infused with subconscious-based techniques. While both groups lost weight, isn't it fabulous that the group who used both strategies lost nearly twice the number of pounds? And the subjects who tapped into the power of their subconscious brains experienced enhanced benefits over time.[3]

SVT can even be a part of helping someone with life-threating habits remain sober. SVT doesn't replace other treatments; it enhances them. Case in point: 261 addicts and alcoholics were admitted to an inpatient treatment program. Then, they were divided into groups. One group got hypnosis training, another group got CBT-based treatment, and a third group was given relaxation training. The results? All three evidence-based models were equally effective—87 percent were sober at a seven-week follow up. But then subjects in the hypnosis group experienced something that the other groups didn't. For the subjects who actually practiced hypnosis by themselves at least four times per week, their sense of serenity and self-worth went up, while their impulsivity and feelings of anger went down.[4]

SVT doesn't replace other treatments; it enhances them.

Imagine people living sensational, sober lives while attending meetings. They continue to practice SVT four times a week. They have more serenity and self-worth. They are less impulsive. Don't you imagine they will be more likely to stay sober year after year than those who didn't add SVT to their program?

TRANCE-FORMING YOUR SENSES

Your subconscious can also perform makeovers on your senses. It's actually quite easy for SVT to help you perceive sugar as being way too sweet. That's because, of all the types of sensations you can create with the subconscious, subtle variation of taste and smell can be easily distorted. With a bit of practice, your subconscious can make diet soda taste disgusting—with a dirt aftertaste and a smell that reminds you of dried urine. Sparkling water and spinach will taste strangely sweet with a few well-placed suggestions. Yes, the subconscious can make you taste or smell things that aren't actually there.

This is all thanks to the subconscious brain's ability to change how you perceive sensations. You could do this slowly and consciously. For example, people who follow a low-sodium diet will eventually perceive processed foods as too salty—but this usually takes about a month. Your subconscious brain can do this in an instant by rewiring the brain's perception system. It's like installing a virus on your own computer—for your advantage and protection.

Remember the study I told you about in Chapter 2, where subjects imagined their hands being burned with their conscious brains and then imagined the same thing via the subconscious? Brain scans of those subjects showed the subconscious—but not the conscious—lighting up those areas of the brain where sensation occurs, thus being able to make sensations that aren't there feel real. People in this group felt their hands being scalded with a hot object, although in actuality nothing happened.

Although visual sensations are by far the most difficult to create subconsciously, research proves it can be done. One hypnosis expert uses a "Santa Claus test" to create visual hallucinations in his patients. As far-fetched as this may sound, this doctor tells patients that when they come out of the subconscious-driven state, they will see the doctor dressed like Santa Claus for a moment—until he says "poof." About 5 percent of his patients witnessed this hallucinatory phenomenon.[5] A recent study used EEGs to measure brain wave activity while studying other visual hallucinations. While hypnotized, subjects were told, "Squares are always red." Later, while they were conscious, this suggestion created visual hallucinations and changed their perception of color.[6] What new network of brain circuitry will you build for yourself?

Perhaps you'll be curious about how to trick your brain's inner pharmacy to release dopamine, serotonin, GABA, and endorphins as if you already have that dream job or are well on your way to losing weight. Cigarettes and sugar aren't the only way to release feel-good hormones; your brain can send them all by itself. Yes, your subconscious brain can actually get you high. And won't it be nice to get a little taste of how good it will feel—especially if the road ahead of you is a long one? The road to losing 200 pounds starts with what you eat for dinner tonight, doesn't it?

SVT FOR HABITS AND HEALTHIER LIVING

Since we can plant positivity in your subconscious, leaving old habits behind will be fairly painless. Taking up new ones may even be surprisingly enjoyable. Any healthy activity—from attending a 12-step meeting to socializing more with friends to gardening—can begin to feel so effortless. And you'll remember how much you enjoy these activities.

Leaving old habits behind will be fairly painless. Taking up new ones may even be surprisingly enjoyable.

This time, the seven steps of SVT will help set you free from unhealthy habits and say hello to healthy ones. I recommend using this practice of SVT at least a few times a week for a month to help build new neural pathways, neutralize triggers, and turn the subconscious vision of the healthy you into your waking, conscious reality.

You'll do step 1 again now as a stand-alone practice as it specifically relates to habits. Then, steps 2 through 7 are done as one seamless practice—as freedom washes over you.

- Step 1: Considering the Conscious

- Step 2: Activating the Subconscious

- Step 3: Revising the Past

- Step 4: Enhancing the Present

- Step 5: Creating the Future

- Step 6: Planting Positivity

- Step 7: Building Bridges

STEP 1: CONSIDERING THE CONSCIOUS

Consider those three pitfall thought patterns you wrote down on page 47. As it relates to any habit preventing you from your best life, is there one pitfall thought pattern that keeps you from sticking to healthy habits? Is there one in particular that is linked to a vice, keeping you tethered to that carton of cigarettes or syrup-drizzled chocolate ice cream?

At the beginning of this chapter, you learned that most unhealthy habits are related to either stress management or sensation seeking. Stress management habits are often linked to anxiety and pitfall thought patterns of paralysis by analysis or polarized thinking. Sensation seeking is sometimes tied to low dopamine and can be related to permanence or pessimism. Perhaps when you review the seven pitfall thought patterns on page 44, you'll see a different pitfall thought pattern tied to your habit. Write down that pitfall thought pattern here:

Type of pitfall thought pattern tied to a habit I want to end: _____

_____

which, to me, is a thought that sounds something like: _____

_____

Now that your conscious brain knows what it needs to change, allow your powerful subconscious brain to figure out how to change it.

It may be helpful to consider the timing of your habits when considering scheduling SVT. If you tend to chain-smoke during your lunch break, perhaps you could retreat to your car at noon and use SVT then. If that pint of ice cream calls to you at 9 P.M., then try SVT at 8 P.M. SVT is a fantastic tool to use as often as needed, and remember, it can be potently combined with other strategies as well.

STEPS 2 THROUGH 7: *SVT FOR HABITS AND HEALTHIER LIVING*

I've included this written SVT script for you to come back to when you're ready to practice without the guided audio tracks. It's also a blueprint for practitioners training in SVT. In a comfortable seated or lying posture, listen to the audio track "SVT for Habits & Healthier Living" (see page 242 for download information) to break unhealthy habits and build healthy ones.

I invite you to begin this practice by allowing the eyes to close as you settle in here . . . as the body finds the most comfortable position to rest. And as you settle here, make any last adjustments if you'd like, resting into this peaceful and pleasurable state. . . . I wonder if you can bring your attention to the place in the body where you feel the most relaxed. You already know how to activate the subconscious, which has always been here conspiring in your favor, so I invite you to begin this journey simply with some mindfulness. Ever so easily invite yourself to simply notice what's on your mind—right here and right now.

And now use the power of your mind's eye to imagine you're watching a parade . . . and this parade is made up of your thoughts . . . your feelings . . . your urges to engage in any habit that's not in alignment with your healthiest and highest self. . . . Isn't it nice to watch them float on by . . . without having to act on them? If you'd like, you could even picture that this parade begins with a grandmaster leading the parade out from your brain through a path out of the ear to a place just in front of you . . . but here you are, watching from the sidelines . . . and feeling so peaceful.

Isn't it so nice to know that you don't have to join the parade . . . no matter where you see the grandmaster leading it? I wonder if that even makes you feel a bit proud of yourself . . . or even more peaceful, perhaps. Many people find it so freeing to know that they don't have to act on these thoughts . . . these feelings . . . these urges . . . you can just watch as the parade passes by.

I wonder if you're even a little amused at how silly this parade can be at times . . . as all our parades tend to be. What do you see? Are people dressed in ridiculous costumes . . . or are there wild animals? I don't know exactly what you'll see in your parade . . . and it really doesn't matter . . .

What matters is if you can bring a lightness to the way you greet your parade. Can you even smile a bit now? Because the train that your subconscious brain is about to show you—and the places that your future self can take you—is far more impressive, isn't it? Oh, the places you will go. Would you like to take a peek? Who would want to board the fast train to nowhere when they could have a first-class ticket to Naples, Nice, or Norway?

*Now pivot your attention to sounds. And invite the ears to notice **three sounds** you're hearing—right here and right now. That's right. It could be interesting to begin with the loudest sound you can perceive in this moment. And now find a noise that's neither loud nor soft—a medium sound. Now, I wonder what's the quietest sound you can hear . . . can you hear your breath? That's right. Perfect.*

*And now invite the eyes to notice **two colors** you can see on the back of the eyelids. The first being directly in front of you . . . and then, on the next inhale, what color can you see near the crown of the head as you roll the eyes up, up, up?*

*On the next exhale, allow the eyes to float down, down, down . . . and just relax the eyes now as you allow any lingering tightness to float away. Yes, that's right. And now I invite you to really feel **one breath**. Allowing the breath to breathe you. Can you feel the breath rocking you? Can you feel the place where the breath feels the most pleasant or the most peaceful? Allow that feel-good or soothing sensation to spread through the brain and body. That's right. Perfect.*

And now I invite you to take the next step by asking the subconscious to help you in the way you need it most today. Isn't it so nice to know that you already have the tools within you to change? By giving yourself this time today, you have already shown that you are honest, open, and willing, haven't you? I wonder what will show up for you today . . . I don't know if it will complement all the tools you already use or if it will help you find some new ones . . . but what I do know is that it will help you find that deep part of you that knows that you are okay . . . that you are innately worthy . . . and as you begin to find pleasure in the simple things, you'll feel this peace and pleasure in ways that are in line with your highest self.

*In just a moment, but not quite yet, I'll invite you to use the power of your mind's eye to see and feel yourself walking down **12 flights of stairs**. Can you see these stairs in front of you? I wonder if you already have a sense that they will lead to that place of sustainable peace and pleasure. Or perhaps they'll take you down to a beautiful beach or to a place where you are surrounded by a soft-white, spiritual light . . . a light that some part of you knows will grow stronger and stronger over time. Visualize those stairs now. What color are they? Are they wood, or are they metal? Is it a spiral staircase, or is it a grand staircase? See yourself standing at the top of that staircase now—that's right—with a feeling that this journey will be exactly what you need today.*

12. *Which foot is taking the first step? Is it the left foot . . . or is it the right? As you feel the body moving down, simply notice a small—or maybe a larger—sense of peace and pleasure washing over you. That's right.*

11. *Feeling the other foot taking that next step on the staircase now. Allowing a deep sense of relaxation . . . and a beautiful sense of surrender . . . to wash over you.*

10. *Stepping down, feeling a sense of serenity wash over you.*

9. *Feeling twice as calm as you were on the floor before.*

8. *Stepping down as the conscious mind lets go of worries. That's right. Good.*

7. *Even deeper now. Perfect.*

6. *Halfway down the staircase now. That's right.*

5. *Stepping down again . . . give yourself this time to take care of yourself.*

4. *Feeling an even deeper sense of serenity wash over you.*

3. *Almost there now. That's right. You're doing so wonderfully already . . . and you've only just begun.*

2. *Next-to-last step. Feeling a bit dreamy now . . .*

1. *Last step. . . . As you allow yourself this time to enjoy this peace . . . this pleasure . . . isn't it so nice to know that these feel-good chemicals are right here . . . within you? And here you are sitting still, and you cultivated this feeling . . . releasing your own inner pharmacy of feel-good chemicals . . . that's right . . . that's right . . . perfect.*

Now that you've felt the body make its way down the staircase, you've probably noticed the brain begin to slow itself down into a state of healing relaxation. In just a moment, you'll feel the body start to float upward as your consciousness begins to expand—as I count up from one to seven. As these two things happen—body floating and consciousness expanding—you may notice an even deeper sense of peace and probably start to feel so good.

As the body begins to float, many people also notice it feels warm—as though you're taking a warm bath or floating in the ocean on a summer day. As you practice this more, you may even find that you lose a sense of time and space. If you'd like, you can even "leave" the physical body for this brief practice during this time you've given yourself. If it feels comfortable, you may wish to see your consciousness actually leaving the physical body as a momentary kind of "out-of-body" experience. If you'd like, you can see your consciousness moving upward toward the sky . . . and returning to the body at the end of the practice or, if you prefer, at any point during it.

Counting now:

1. *Body float.*

2. *Consciousness moving upward and expanding so that it's now larger than the body.*

3. *Body becoming lighter and warmer.*

4. *Consciousness moving upward and expanding even more so that it fills the room.*

5. *Body becoming almost weightless now.*

6. *Consciousness so elevated and expanded that it's joining with the universe . . . feeling a great white light glowing all around you.*

7. *So deep and so relaxed. Perfect.*

Now, in your mind's eye . . . I invite you to visualize a guide . . . and see someone who always makes you feel supported and loved. It could be your mother, your partner, your dog, or your sponsor. I don't know who it will be for you, but I do know that this is the image of a person who helps you through this journey. And when you picture this person, you will find yourself with an inner sense of serenity in your heart. That's right . . . you can feel that, can't you? Because, no matter what, you are never truly alone. You know that, don't you? Can you feel this person's presence? Can you feel that love that will always be with you?

In just a moment, but not quite yet, we'll ask your subconscious to rewind the tape to a time in your past . . . a time when you used a habit as a less-than-ideal way to cope with everything you were going through. I wonder if it was to deal with stress . . . because you were desperate for a feeling of peace. Or I wonder if it was to deal with boredom or depression . . . because you just wanted to feel good. Either way, it's so nice to know that the subconscious has the power to rewire and release you as it forms new pathways, isn't it? Now I'm going to ask your subconscious to go as far back as you need to go—to a time when you used a habit in an unhealthy way. For this first time you see this scene from your past, just allow the scene to play . . . with you as the viewer—just like you're watching a show on TV. I wonder if the subconscious will help show you see this scene in a way that feels new in some way . . .

As I count backward from three to one, the eyes will relax, and the eyes will flutter left and right just a bit more now. I'll invite you to flutter the eyes back and forth—left and right—just a bit more. Pressing play on that scene or scenes from the past—you and this habit that wasn't in line with your healthiest, happiest, and highest self . . . and allowing the eyes to flutter a bit now left and right on three . . . two . . . one [left-right-left-right audio tones].

Now inhale on the count of three: one, two, three. Exhale on the count of six: one, two, three, four, five, six. While there may be a bit of tension, I wonder if you can notice the place where can feel at ease. . . . After all, you're here now, taking care of your-

self . . . and as I count from one to five, the subconscious brain will spread this ease to the rest of the mind, body, and spirit: one, two, three, four, five. That's right. Perfect.

In just a moment, I'm going to have you play that scene again. This time, you're going to see a split screen. On the left, you'll see the same scene you just saw—that cigarette, that pint of ice cream, you biting your nails . . . or whatever habit is robbing from you the health or wealth you deserve. On the right side of the screen, the subconscious brain is going to highlight something the conscious brain may have missed: the strengths you already have within you . . . and have always had. You were using a coping mechanism to deal with stress or to feel good, but what if you were strong enough or good enough all along?

Most of us are so hard on ourselves all the time. So allow your generous and kind subconscious brain to highlight what's right within you. If you can see that you have already accomplished so much, you can remember your inherent self-worth. If you can know how much you have gotten through, then you know that you'll be okay. And perhaps you could even see what was motivating the habit that was robbing you of your truest self . . . if you were so stressed that you turned to that cigarette or so alone that you turned to those salty caramels. I wonder if you . . . or the person who you brought on this journey with you . . . could find some compassion for that younger version of yourself . . . for the you who was struggling or sad or stressed. Invite the subconscious to show you something.

In just a moment, you'll see a split screen. The left side of the screen will be the same scene you just played a moment ago . . . on the right side, you'll see your inherent goodness, your inherent self-worth, and what you needed . . . with a healthy dose of compassion.

Now, pressing play on that split screen, see the scene unfold— the scene as you saw it a moment ago on the left and the same scene unfolding with something kinder, more confident, or gen-

tler on the right . . . that part of you that realizes that you were calm enough, good enough this whole time . . . as you allow the eyes to flutter now on three . . . two . . . one . . . [left-right-left-right audio tones].

Now inhale on the count of three: one, two, three. Exhale on the count of six: one, two, three, four, five, six. And bring your attention to a place in the body where you feel a bit of serenity . . . that's right. That's right. Perfect.

Letting go of the split screen now, now see just one screen. In just a moment, you'll open up that advanced editing software so you can see that film being projected again. I wonder what the subconscious brain would like to do to in that one scene. What would you like to do to transform vices into victory? This time, you have the power to press delete on any behavior, any trigger, any naysaying voice—whether it was someone else's or your own. . . . When you do, it will be so empowering, won't it? You could see your past self saying yes to all those healthier choices that support you. Or perhaps you'd like to get rid of that scene completely. Simply press delete if you'd like. In just a moment, the power of the subconscious brain will start to set you free. And again, notice—in this wonderfully relaxed state— where in your body you feel the most relaxed.

So now pressing play on this scene again . . . but also making any changes to this scene, editing or deleting it in any way that supports that healthiest version of you, as you allow the eyes to flutter now on three . . . two . . . one . . . [left-right-left-right audio tones].

Now inhale on the count of three: one, two, three. Exhale on the count of six: one, two, three, four, five, six. What did you see? And what did that feel like? Now, as I count from one to five, imagine that the subconscious is spreading this feeling to every part of the brain and body . . . so that this pathway is the new default way to be. After all, habits are habits because they are familiar . . . so help the brain become familiar with a new way of life now . . . show your brain something better. Try it on. See it. Feel it. Create the pathway. That's right one . . . two . . . three . . . four . . . five . . . that's right. Perfect.

And now allow the subconscious brain to fast-forward to present day. Isn't it so interesting that the subconscious brain has already begun to set you free from habits—the ones preventing you from living the healthy, incredible life you were born to live? Some part of you knows this already. . . . What made you realize this? Was it the way the subconscious brain helped you to connect the dots, or was it the compassion you cultivated for yourself? Just take a moment here to notice what feels different now. I don't know if the difference will be a subtle one or a significant one, but you will notice something right now or tomorrow afternoon. Isn't it so interesting that in this moment, you may even be able to find one or two pieces of evidence that a new light has already been lit somewhere deep within you? With honesty, openness, and willingness, you already have the tools to set yourself free.

And in this moment, you feel as though you're floating on a pink cloud . . . one that is bringing you peace and health from within. And this pink cloud is one that lasts and will stay with you forever . . . transforming from pink to purple to white. . . . You also know—right here and right now—that you are so much stronger than you realize. You no longer need to use avoidance or self-medication . . . because you already have the tools and an inner pharmacy of feel-good chemicals . . . and an endless supply of ways to manifest health at your disposal.

Now imagine that you are a computer hacker . . . and as you go in and open the operating system of your brain, can you see those programs that have wired you for habits? In just a moment, we're going to short-circuit those negative habits. From now on, you will become completely blind to them . . . and your senses will conspire only for your health . . . rather than noticing or recognizing triggers. . . . Also, we'll do the opposite for anything that's in line with your highest self. We will turn up the sensitivity that you have for any opportunity to create health for yourself, so your brain will be like a hypersensitive smoke alarm that goes off whenever you turn the oven on. Turn off the alarm for unhealthy habits; turn on the alarm for health. That's right. Hack your own system. And forget that you have done this after this practice is over . . . so that this process becomes even more effortless.

And now let's cross wires so that your favorite unhealthy taste or smell becomes completely repulsive. Like a phone operator who patches a wire over to the wrong line, open up the box to your brain's senses. Can you see that box? Now can you see the wire for that one sense that you crave? The smell of freshly baked cookies? Is it that first sip of a diet soda . . . and the way the bubbles hit your tongue? The way you love to hit the pack of cigarettes on your arm or palm? Now match that sense to the same sense—smell to smell, taste to taste—but ask your subconscious to find something in your sense memory that you find repulsive. If the smell of cookies is your trigger, perhaps you ask your subconscious to tell you it's the smell of rotting fish. If the taste of soda is what you crave, perhaps your subconscious changes it to the taste of urine. Now see your brain crossing the wires. See them in the same place in your mind's eye. As you bring forth both sense memories, fuse them together—cookies and fish, soda and urine . . . or whatever your subconscious would like to create here . . . and since the subconscious is so suggestible, from this point on, you will be reminded of this repulsive taste or smell whenever you encounter your unhealthy habit trigger. . . . I wonder when you'll notice this disgusting smell now that you've planted this suggestion in the subconscious. It'll be like trying not to think of a pink elephant if I tell you not to think of a pink elephant . . . now that idea is there. And I wonder when you'll notice the faint smell of burning hair, flesh, or urine in that diet soda, ice cream, or cigarette. After all, you do know that all those vices are toxic chemicals, don't you?

So perhaps the subconscious is helping you to perceive things for what they really are . . . and the delicious, divine, nutritious foods that come from nature will taste better than ever before to you . . . and activities that are healthy or spiritually fulfilling for you will feel effortless. After all, they are in line with your true nature of health and healing.

And now the subconscious is going to help you fast-forward your life. Try on the new you, the healthy you . . . because what you're really doing is trading short-term pennies for long-term millions, aren't you? Wouldn't it be so wonderful to see the destination? To try this on? To feel it? The future serene, healthy you . . . and since time and space begins to fade away in the next few moments, you'll also see everything that you need to do in the weeks and even years to follow. See it all unfold step-by-step. I wonder if those steps include more spin classes, salads, or a sponsor for you. Feel it happening—right here, right now. Whatever it is that you see, these specific, measurable, achievable, relevant, and time-sensitive goals will unfold—and this will allow the conscious brain to go out and create them. And you'll take it day by day. That's right. Seeing it all so clearly now. Can you even turn the dial up on how good it all feels? That's right. And how healthy and happy you are . . . oh yes . . . that's fine . . . perfect.

Deepen this state now one more time so the positive messages you are about to hear will be planted deeply in the subconscious brain as I count backward from three to one: three . . . two . . . one . . . that's right. You have done so much here to take care of yourself today, haven't you? To be happier . . . to be healthier . . . to tap back into that highest self. If you're as sick as your secrets, then just being here is you taking care of yourself and being rigorously honest, isn't it? And all the changes you've already made will begin to unfold in a way that feels simple and effortless. I'm not sure if you'll notice it in the way you talk to others . . . or perhaps a change in that parade of thoughts or urges. I wonder if it will be tomorrow when you notice that something has changed—or if it will be sometime next Tuesday afternoon. You are already a bit more free from the vices that held you back, aren't you? Isn't that such an incredible feeling to notice where you have already begun to make a change and how new, healthy behaviors will begin to replace old habits that were holding you back? Yes, your highest self will unfold in effortless ways every day, and this will help your future self to go to some really fabulous places.

Now it's time to build a bridge that will help you connect everything you have done here during this practice—so that you can take it with you into your waking life. The first part of building this bridge involves a button. I wonder: What were the three best lessons, "aha" moments, insights, or feelings you felt here? Visualize them now . . . and send them down into the index finger of your dominant hand. And really feel them growing—turning them up now, growing and glowing with intensity. Can you feel it? That's right. Now rub the tip of that index finger with that thumb. There. You've just built a button for yourself. In your waking, everyday life—whenever you need a little piece of what you've created here—all you need to do is to push that button. All the peace, all the feel-good feelings, all the "aha" moments will come flooding back. Isn't it so nice that you have what it takes to "get high," so to speak—on wholeness, on healthy living, on spiritual friendship, on love, on faith—here within you, at any time? Those are natural highs that will last . . . and ones that just keep getting better with time.

Second, gather any residual stuff you'd like to get rid of—resentment and rage, negativity and naysaying voices. Now visualize a balloon tied to your nondominant index finger. Can you see it? See that balloon being blown up as you fill it with the "hot air" of habits that are not serving your highest self. Many people may even notice that this finger will begin to lift on its own. Isn't that interesting? One last moment here—see if there's anything else you'd like to put in that balloon. That's right. And now rub that thumb against your nondominant index finger to untie that balloon. In your mind's eye, see that balloon float far, far away. Can you see it becoming so small, so tiny now? Follow it until it's gone. And whenever you notice any of this "stuff" that does not serve your highest, healthiest self, all you need to do is put it into this balloon that's tied to your nondominant index finger. Then, rub your thumb to untie the string . . . and let it all go. You're free.

And now see yourself walking back up those stairs that brought you here to this place of serenity and healing—knowing you can return here as often as you'd like. Stepping up and becoming twice as awake on every step. And as you do, coming back to your waking, everyday state . . . as consciousness returns to the body . . . with a renewed sense of excitement to create that future self you saw.

1. *Stepping up. Feel yourself becoming alert now.*

2. *Another step up. Become more awake, feeling hopeful.*

3. *Perhaps giving a wiggle to your fingers and your toes.*

4. *That's right. Up and activated. Feeling your consciousness returning to your body. So present. So alive.*

5. *Twice as energized and alert as you were on the step before.*

6. *Stepping up again.*

7. *Awake and alert . . . consciousness fully back in your body now.*

8. *That's right. So energized.*

9. *Stepping up again and feeling ready to create that future self.*

10. *Feeling your body ascend.*

11. *Almost there.*

12. *Eyes open. Awake. Refreshed.*

To ensure you're fully conscious again, look around the room and name aloud 10 items you see, take a walk around the block, listen to some upbeat music, or do 25 jumping jacks.

CHAPTER 11

SVT for Healing Your Body, Pain, and Elusive Conditions

The subconscious brain is truly powerful. Did you know hypnosis was the go-to anesthesia for physicians in 19th-century India before the discovery of ether? Hypnosis was one of the first forms of mindbody medicine. The subconscious brain is so potent in its pain-relieving potential that it was even used for limb amputations.[1]

Isn't it fascinating that the subconscious brain has the power to change bodily processes? It can reduce or eliminate the need for drugs. What if I told you your subconscious could actually tell your body to bleed less? It's true: if I used SVT to plant positivity before surgery and told your subconscious you would bleed less during surgery, your body would lose less blood than the body of someone who didn't use SVT. That's what one study proved.[2]

I wonder what physical goal SVT could help you with? Would you like to heal your body—or optimize it? Would you like to boost your immune system? Whether you're fighting stage IV cancer or facing flu season, you can combine SVT with existing treatments or use it as a preventative tonic.

Perhaps you'd like to use SVT to help you deal with pain. Did you know your subconscious brain can effectively help you with anything from the most minor, temporary ache to severe, chronic pain? Wouldn't it be incredible to find relief without drugs?

And if you've been diagnosed with an elusive condition such as migraines, fibromyalgia, IBS, chronic fatigue syndrome, restless legs syndrome, overactive bladder, painful bladder syndrome, post-Lyme disease syndrome, eczema, multiple sclerosis, or any other condition that a) doesn't respond all that well to modern medicine and/or b) is exacerbated by stress, I imagine you'd love to find something that would bring relief.

First, brain. Then, body.

You're probably starting to understand the sheer power of the subconscious brain when focused in the direction of mindbody healing. Other treatments, like behavioral modification, work on a surface level, as they help you avoid triggers, and pain pills temporarily numb pain. The subconscious works on a much deeper, more profound level. That's why I use SVT to treat pain, optimize immune function, and heal elusive syndromes.

I have found that SVT truly excels in the areas where modern Western medicine has little or nothing to offer—because SVT tends to work with complex conditions that are ruled by the brain (where belief and hope are powerful medicines). Yes, plenty of prescription medications are available, but you often get a small improvement for a high cost and lots of side effects. (Plus, some of those improvements may simply be the power of your subconscious brain believing that the medication is working. See discussion of the placebo effect in Chapter 1.) On the other hand, SVT is an inexpensive, drug-free tool you can use as much as you'd like. It comes with a long list of side benefits (enhanced immune function, a feeling of peace, increased motivation to engage in healthy behaviors) instead of side effects. After numerous medications provided them with no answers, people I've treated with these conditions have often reported they find SVT to be nothing short of miraculous.

Now, perhaps you'd still prefer some modern anesthesia if you need major surgery—great, me too. (On the other hand, I have watched a video of a patient who had major surgery and only "went under" with the power of his subconscious brain.) I wonder if you'd be interested in using your subconscious brain to need less anesthesia and feel decreased post-operative pain. Studies have shown the power of subconscious brain–based techniques to accelerate post-surgical wound healing[3] and help patients with cancer to reduce nausea and vomiting.[4]

One study divided patients undergoing thyroid surgery into two groups. Twenty patients "went under" with general anesthesia, and twenty patients got hypnosedation, a combination of hypnosis, local anesthesia, and light sedation. The hypnosedation group experienced less inflammation, less post-operative pain, and less post-operative fatigue than the general anesthesia group.[5]

Breast cancer survivor Kelly Painter entered a newer trial using hypnosedation at MD Anderson Cancer Center to have her tumor surgically removed in 2017. She reported, "It took a little longer than a traditional surgery because they had to numb the area with lidocaine. But even so, I was in the operating room at 8:30 A.M., out of surgery by 11:30 A.M., and out of the hospital by 12:15 P.M. I never even really felt hypnotized, and the worst pain I felt was a little pinch. It was mostly just pressure. . . . And I didn't have to take any pain medicine afterward."[6]

Or consider something as common as painful menstrual cramps. One study randomly divided 50 nursing students with painful cramps into two groups. One received ibuprofen for three menstrual cycles and then no medication for the following three cycles. The second group received hypnosis. Not surprisingly, the medication group only experienced pain relief for the three cycles when they took the ibuprofen and had no significant pain reduction for the following three cycles. The hypnosis group experienced a significant reduction in pain for all six cycles.[7] Remember, ibuprofen is one of over-the-counter drugs that the FDA warned may spike risk of heart attack and stroke—even in short-term use. If there were no alternative for someone in pain, the risk may warrant the benefit. But this study shows that a risk-free alternative does exist, and it uses your subconscious brain.

INTEGRATIVE VISUALIZATION

When it comes to cancer, autoimmune conditions, chronic pain, and elusive conditions, throwing a bunch of prescription pain pills at someone is like throwing water on a grease fire. So it's important to integrate SVT into a holistic treatment plan. As you already know, SVT incorporates many strategies, including CBT, mindfulness, hypnosis, bilateral stimulation, and guided visualization, into one easy-to-use, at-home tool. If your well-being is at stake, it may also mean pulling out all the stops. Cut gluten or dairy. Limit your toxin exposure, especially if environmental toxins have triggered an autoimmune condition. Pairing a liposomal glutathione supplement with SVT is just one example of a strategy that may be used for detoxification. If the brain is damaged from injury or stroke, hydrogen can be used to help in the healing process. A far infrared sauna is another evidence-based, drug-free possibility that I frequently recommend. They improve the quality of life for those with diabetes,[8] and just eight sessions of side effect–free infrared sauna also led to a clinically significant reduction in pain and stiffness in people living with rheumatoid arthritis.[9] Wouldn't it be interesting to do a session of SVT while you were in a far infrared sauna?

Tests & Tools

I also recommend the latest in evidence-based care, including genetic testing and a neurotransmitter panel, to determine what may be causing or exacerbating an elusive condition or chronic pain. Genetic testing is empowering. You may have inherited an inability to convert certain B vitamin precursors into the forms usable by the brain and body. Without these usable forms, you may have neurotransmitter deficiencies that affect pain, anxiety, and mood.

Audio-visual entrainment (AVE) can also deepen SVT or be used as a stand-alone tool to help with certain elusive conditions. For example, a fast beta wave AVE session may help someone struggling with chronic fatigue syndrome feel more energetic (see page 242). Find out more about AVE on my website, drmikedow.com.

If you're undergoing chemo for stage IV cancer, working with a functional medicine practitioner to discover the root of your illness, or undergoing individual psychotherapy (whether the practitioner is trained in SVT or another model of psychotherapy), I say to you: that's wonderful. SVT is a tool that supports all these integrative strategies.

So let's take a look at how the science of the immune system, pain, and elusive conditions, along with the subconscious, can come together to help you improve any of these conditions.

Boosting your immunity

I already mentioned one group of people who can use SVT to boost their immune system: people surviving cancer. (Did you notice my choice of words when I said "surviving cancer"? I'm already beginning to speak to the powerful, intimate way your subconscious brain works with your immune system.) But not only cancer thrivers can benefit from an immune-system boost.

The common cold, herpes, HIV, HPV, eczema, breakups, losing your job, traveling, or just the stress of everyday life all take a toll on the immune system. In fact, I can't think of anyone who couldn't benefit from a stronger immune system, can you?

Our world is becoming more polluted, and exposure to toxins can "turn on" genes for autoimmune conditions, where your body attacks its own tissues. Multiple sclerosis, Hashimoto's disease, lupus, psoriasis, arthritis; the list goes on and on. According to the NIH, more than 23 million Americans are now living with an auto-immune condition. These conditions tend to be more common in women—possibly because of the complex interplay of estrogen and progesterone, and the way those hormones interact with the immune system. Exposure to asbestos, radiation, solvents, and the gluten-rich American diet are all noted culprits. And even more Americans may have "preautoimmunity."[10] A 2012 study found that over 30 million Americans have autoantibodies, a marker of autoimmune disease, which are often measurable years before an autoimmune condition surfaces.[11] Just one example: exposure to mercury in fish leads to a rise in autoantibodies in the blood of pregnant women and their fetuses.[12]

Most drugs that aim to treat autoimmune conditions make a fundamental mistake: they treat the immune system and the brain as two distinct and independent systems and view disease as a simple cause-and-effect process that must be cured—a biolog-ical model. On the other hand, SVT believes in coherence: your brain and immune system are actually intertwined and are trying to serve a common purpose.[13] SVT operates on the principle that disease (the distance from ease) is the result of complex, interre-lated systems that have gone awry and that can only be healed through a bio-psycho-social-spiritual or holistic model of care. The biological model is akin to one person trying to take apart and reassemble a car's engine with just one giant hammer in the mechanic's toolbelt. The bio-psycho-social-spiritual model is a team of mechanics working to rebuild that engine with advanced, computer-guided tools.

While we're still in the infancy of understanding autoimmune conditions, researchers believe that the brain and immune system communicate via the limbic-hypothalamic-pituitary pathway.[14] So if your immune system and brain are working together (albeit in complex ways), then perhaps they are trying to help you when they perceive a threat: that mercury you ate or those fumes you just inhaled.

How could an awful autoimmune disease be your body's way of helping you? Well, think of a bear hibernating—that's how he survives a terribly harsh winter. In many ways, this is exactly what our world has become: harsh, toxic, and stressful. Now, let's look at human beings diagnosed with chronic fatigue syndrome (CFS). A groundbreaking 2016 study found that of the 612 metabolites the researchers examined, 80 percent were lower in those with CFS. Essentially, their bodies had gone into a human form of hibernation. But unlike animals that hibernate, people with CFS have cells that get stuck in an energy-conserving state—and don't know how to wake back up.[15] This landmark study sheds light on autoimmune conditions: your brain and immune system think they are helping you. They identify all those toxins or a virus coming in and see: *Threat! Protect yourself!* They will react with either *fight* or *flight/freeze* responses. A healthy response is to *fight*—attack the bad guys, save the good guys. If you have an autoimmune disease, your cells get confused. Imagine a football team who randomly swaps jerseys. Now your immune system begins tackling its own players—it's *fighting*. Or, in the case of CFS, your immune system exhibits a more *flight/freeze* response and shuts down. A *flight/freeze* response should be used when you determine that you'd lose the fistfight with the guy at the bar who's twice your size. Better to either scram or play dead. Save your energy for a match you'd win. In CFS, this *flight/freeze* response isn't strategic because when there is a match your immune system you could win, it's still nowhere to be found.

Cue SVT. Could your subconscious brain help with these incredibly elusive, difficult-to-treat conditions? Good news—the answer is yes.

The immune boost provided by the subconscious brain is so powerful, it can be measured in your blood. Remember that study I told you about in Chapter 2? It divided medical students into two groups as they were facing their exams. One learned how to practice self-hypnosis, the other didn't. The group who activated their subconscious experienced a major enhancement in immune function. Blood tests revealed strong differences in measuring two white blood cell markers used to assess immune function. The markers decreased for the group without hypnosis, but the more the other students used the hypnosis tape at home, the more their T-lymphocyte markers' numbers went up.[16] Imagine how SVT could boost your immunity during another stressful time in your life, such as a round of chemo or the daily grind of being a working parent.

SVT speaks to a complex, interrelated set of systems that caused the symptoms of autoimmune disorders in the first place. You have to go deep and affect systems and pathways. You have to tell your cells what to do. As far-fetched as that may sound, remember that study I just told you about: the subconscious brain can make the body bleed less—something the conscious brain can't do. By the same token, SVT can achieve results that are nothing short of remarkable. And like a crazy man who talks to his dogs as though they speak English (I am that man; call me crazy), you can talk to your cells, tissues, organs, and systems and tell them to wake up, heal, spare the good cells, target malignant ones, or anything else you'd like them to do. An immune system that is underactive can wake up, or one that's hyperactive can get turned down.

You can talk to your cells, tissues, organs, and systems and tell them to wake up, heal, spare the good cells, target malignant ones, or anything else you'd like them to do.

The proof? Consider the following study results:

- In this day and age, it would seem silly to suggest mindbody medicine to rid your body of unsightly warts, caused by the class of viruses known as HPV. Just head to the drug store and pick up some salicylic acid, a proven treatment. One randomized controlled study included a placebo group taking salicylic acid and an experimental group using hypnosis for the treatment of warts. The hypnosis focused on imagery suggesting that the warts would tingle, grow warm, shrink, and dissolve away. After six weeks, hypnosis was the most effective treatment for shrinking the warts.[17]

- In a skin study, 38 subjects with itchy skin patches (similar to what you may see in someone with eczema, which, by the way, was classified as an autoimmune condition in 2014[18]) were led through a session that combined hypnosis, cognitive-behavioral strategies, imagination, and visualization. Of the 38 subjects, 32 were able to decrease the size of their skin patches.[19]

- Another study on patients with rheumatoid arthritis (RA) divided them into three groups. One group got hypnosis—they "talked" to the underlying condition and immune system via the subconscious brain. A second group learned relaxation skills. A third group received no treatment. When measuring their leukocytes, researchers discovered that the hypnosis group outperformed the other groups, and the immune boost they received, as well as the reduction in joint pain, swelling, and stiffness, got even better as the subjects continued to practice hypnosis at home.[20]

Since SVT can work synergistically with other strategies to heal your body through its complex connection with the brain, you can see improvement above and beyond what other options offer. Wouldn't you love to find out how much more improvement your own body can make? In the United Kingdom in the 1990s, one researcher published three case studies on people with CFS. All the patients had some symptom improvement, but the researcher noted that hypnosis should be combined with CBT for optimal results.[21] As you know, that's exactly what SVT does: combines the power of the subconscious with CBT-based strategies.

CBT isn't the only treatment that SVT enhances. It can also combat side effects and rebuild the body's energy. People undergoing cancer treatments experience the same core symptom as many people with autoimmune conditions: fatigue. And 40 percent of people who undergo radiation may experience fatigue for up to a year after treatment.[22] A 2014 study published in the *Journal of Clinical Oncology* divided women undergoing radiation for breast cancer into two groups. Both groups received the same amount of time with a therapist. Patients in the first group received supportive and empathic comments. Patients in group two learned the basics of CBT and then went through brief, 15-minute hypnosis practices. The results: hypnosis with CBT outperformed the other group and was effective at reducing both general and muscular fatigue. And even though the hypnosis was not ongoing, the superior boost in energy in the hypnosis with CBT group was still evident when the researchers went back to assess both groups six months later.[23]

Whether you're a cancer thriver, thyroid trooper, or chronic fatigue fighter, I wonder if all this clinical and concrete data will allow your own conscious brain to let down its guard so we can actually put SVT to work on your immune system. The more the conscious brain lets go, the more the subconscious will be set free to weave its imaginative, immune-boosting spells.

PAIN, PAIN, GO AWAY

Wouldn't it be wonderful to tap into the power of your subconscious brain to transform tension into carefree comfort and pain into ease? I probably don't have to convince anyone with chronic pain how nice it would be to find relief without needing to rely on addictive drugs. Chronic pain can be excruciating and "crazy-making"—at least that's how I'd describe it when I had a bulging disc that sent shooting pain from my neck down to my arm. Oh, how I wish my younger self knew how to activate his subconscious brain to ease that pain. While I avoided addictive pain pills, the pain persisted through my treatment of physical therapy and cold, hard patience for two long years.

I see what pain pills have done to the lives of people I've treated. I've heard heart-wrenching stories of housewives becoming heroin addicts and doting dads hooked on Demerol. Bulging discs, burns, phantom limb pain—with those and many other syndromes, a brain scan shows the pain the patient perceives. And it can be bad—*really* bad. So yes, I know and understand why people turn to pain pills: they just want relief, especially when they don't see any true long-term solution to their pain otherwise. Don't we all want to be free from pain? But then, you get hooked. And when you try to stop, the pain is worse than when it started.

And it's not just people who are popping OxyContin or begging ER docs for Dilaudid. What about all of us who pop "harmless" over-the-counter pain relievers for minor aches and pains? Those are fine, right? Maybe not. As noted earlier, in 2015, the FDA strengthened its original 2005 warning that these over-the-counter pain relievers increase the risk of heart attack and stroke—even with short-term use. While certainly not in the same category as prescription opioids, even over-the-counter pain pills are not without their risks. If you end up having a heart attack or a stroke as the result of using anti-inflammatories, that's no minor "side effect."

With that in mind, what if SVT could deliver the same results—without the risk of heart attack, stroke, or addiction? SVT begins with a fundamental shift in the concept of pain itself. It moves away from the cause-and-effect, biological model of disease (the philosophy behind pain killers), which asks, On a scale of 0 to 10, how bad is your pain? That model then tries to medicate the pain down to zero. SVT operates from a bio-psycho-social-spiritual model of disease, asking, On a scale of 0 to 10, how much ease do you feel now? Where do you feel it the most? And what helps you to turn up that ease? I wonder if you can turn that dial up now . . .

you can, can't you? If you've ever had any sort of muscular tension, you can increase it just by tensing up, can't you? And if you can use the brain to dial something up in the body, doesn't that also mean you can dial it down?

Can you spot the difference between those two lines of thought? Instead of focusing on the negative, SVT looks for (and then turns up) the positive. It also shows people how to tap into the brain's own inner pharmacy of meds. When it comes to pain and the brain, that's vital. If we look at how pain operates in the brain and body, this will help you understand why flipping the script transforms pain to ease, just one of the many strategies of SVT and one of the many unique skills of the subconscious brain.

Earlier EEG research looked at how pain would light up one or two areas of the brain. More recent studies have shown that pain is really the interaction between a number of systems within the brain and body.[24] Interestingly, some of the parts of the brain that are most lit up by pain—like the anterior cingulate cortex and prefrontal cortex—are the same areas identified in Chapters 2 and 4 as parts that you can either turn down or rewire with the subconscious brain.

So here's how pain works: you touch a cup filled with hot water, and that hot cup sends a message from the skin on your hand up your spinal cord to your brain. The sensation is unpleasant—and it's there to keep you safe. Your brain tells the body, "Drop it!" And hopefully, the hand listens.

Imagine if you *didn't* feel pain. Children born with congenital insensitivity to pain (CIP) injure themselves by chewing their own tongues. Not surprisingly, they also have an increased risk of premature death. So yes, pain is there to *keep you alive*. In its most basic form, pain is information that's telling you something: Don't touch that hot cup. Move away from that fire.

More complex associations take longer to change, like the association between chronic pain and obesity. The pain is your body telling you, "Move more and change the way you eat." A sedentary lifestyle and standard American diet create inflammation, which will lead to more pain. Of course, changing this takes a lot longer than moving a hand away from a hot cup. It also creates a paradox, because the changes you need to make now feel more difficult than they were before. You're 100 pounds overweight, and a doctor tells you to exercise more. You think, *Why did I let myself get this big?* That hopelessness creates more pain, and you're caught in a downward spiral.

The antidote: SVT. The subconscious brain isn't going to let you berate yourself; it's going to help you see the change unfold—and then manifest daily—so you can feel more carefree comfort. SVT can be one of the many tools on a weight loss journey.

Now, chronic pain is interesting as it isn't a simple one-way street from your body up your spinal cord to your brain. This may shed light on pain conditions that are based in the brain. Let's say you lose weight, but the chronic pain persists. Sometimes, pain is *not* telling you that something needs to change. Many pain conditions are essentially a false alarm. If that alarm is a signal that a major organ is failing, call 911. That's a job for a surgeon. But it may be that there is nothing really wrong in the body. It's a false alarm—one with its roots in the brain. As these roots are planted deep within the brain, SVT can be helpful in accessing them.

Whenever you encounter something that hurts you—like that hot cup—a signal travels up your spinal cord to your brain. The more signals travel, the more pathways become etched. Thus, pain tends to beget more pain. (By the same token, comfort tends to create more comfort.) The threshold for a pain signal lowers the more it's fired—a hot cup now feels scalding hot. Electrical signals in the brain get in on the action, encouraging feedback loops in the same direction. Yale neurobiologist David McCormick put it this way: "It's like asking whether the roar of the crowd in the football stadium also influences you to cheer as well. And in turn, your cheering encourages others to cheer along with you."[25]

This whole "pain feedback loop" is also influenced by your expectations. Imagine you are in an experiment. The subject in the laboratory just before you tells you, "That cup just burned my skin off!" When it's your turn to hold that cup, what do you think happens to your perception of pain? That person's opinion has told your brain to send signals down to your hand, turning up the pain signal that is about to travel up from your hand to your brain.

Emotion is another player in the pain feedback loop. Imagine you also received a text message just before you walked into the lab. What if someone had sent you something that made you laugh? Or what if your boss just told you that you were getting fired? Would that affect how you perceived pain? The answer is yes, because a relationship exists between your mood and pain. Chronic pain can often make people feel hopeless and depressed, which of course makes pain worse. The subconscious brain is fantastic at interrupting this downward spiral by interrupting these feedback loops. You already know how SVT can boost your mood. The more you improve your mood, the more SVT will create bodily comfort.

However, because SVT is so effective at transforming pain into cool, carefree comfort, I always recommend that you first report any major symptoms to a health care professional who can help rule out major disease. Since pain is information designed to keep you safe, you don't want to turn off signals that could be a warning sign. But most people with chronic pain, fibromyalgia, or migraines have already been told that everything is fine—it's that false alarm again.

Important Note about Pain

Before using SVT to relieve acute or chronic pain, always report your pain symptoms to a health care professional first to determine if you have a disease or injury. Remember, pain is one way your brain and body give you information. Once cleared, you may then confidently use SVT to change the false alarms, pathways, and feedback loops that contribute to pain.

So how does SVT perform all this alchemy? Several ways. Perhaps the simplest way the subconscious brain does this is to slow down the brain—from fast beta brain waves into those slow, dreamy theta brain waves. As you already know, boosting theta brain waves reduces anxiety and can turn on that "delete" button to dissolve traumatic memories. Slowing down the brain is also effective at transforming pain into comfort, since fast beta brain waves have been associated with both acute and chronic pain.[26]

One head-to-head study compared four drug-free treatments for pain against a placebo group. Of those tools, only hypnosis and meditation led to clinically significant reductions in pain. As you know, hypnosis and meditation are both elements of SVT. And between hypnosis and meditation, hypnosis was the better at slowing the brain—less beta, more theta. The gamma brain wave was also boosted by hypnosis.[27] While you already know gamma as the "aha" moment brain wave, it's also involved in the way our brains process pain.

SVT tinkers with all sorts of other processes. As it plants positivity and shifts your attention to how you transform tightness into comfort, it's also tinkering with the feedback loop. SVT can get into the brain to change the messages that are moving from your hand up to your brain or from your brain down to your hand. SVT alters your expectations and diverts your attention to more positive sensations. It's like a kind nurse tapping your left side as the doctor slides a needle into the right arm. That was easy. SVT also tinkers with top-down processing (see Chapter 8), helping you overrule incoming information. Remember that study where the subjects heard, *Squares are always red*? What if someone with headaches heard, *Sensations in the head are simply pressure*. You've just reclassified it. *That's not pain; it's pressure*. You can use your subconscious as the brain's own Icy Hot, reclassifying that burning sensation into a warming one . . . and then into a cool, menthol-like feeling. There's still a sensation there, but your brain categorizes it differently.

By weaving in guided visualization, rehearsal, and CBT, the integrative strategy of SVT allows you to see any big-picture changes happening. The pitfall thought pattern of permanence is banished, and you have hope. You can see your future, and maybe this puts a half-smile on your face during tomorrow's physical therapy session, helping you to push yourself 20 minutes longer—which, in the long run, helps you to feel more comfortable and carefree.

All this brain magic (science) may also have something to do with another 2015 discovery: people with chronic pain have activated glial cells. Scientists used to think glial cells—these are the most abundant cells in your brain[28]—were just fillers in the brain; *glia* is Greek for glue. Since they don't generate the electrical impulses involved in mood and mental illness, they have been largely ignored. If neurons were the star players, glial cells were the water boys. Now it's believed glial cells may be able to remodel circuits in the brain, unplug synapses related to chronic pain and depression, and play a role in regulating neurotransmitter levels. While more research is needed, it could be that the subconscious brain partially weaves its healing magic through the advanced mechanisms by which it interacts with glial cells. After all, the subconscious taps into imagination, and one neuroscientist has called glial cells the "source of the imagination."[29]

But what about something like debilitating neuropathic pain—such as the kind that can result after a car crash? What if you could supercharge the power of the subconscious brain with virtual reality for extreme cases where rapid pain relief is needed? One study divided patients experiencing acute pain into two groups. The first group donned virtual reality (VR) glasses that took them into a beautiful snowy world. The second did the same while activating their subconscious brains. The subjects in this group heard: *Imagine you will see yourself functioning very well. You will be happy. Your pain will be well controlled. You will be sleeping well, and you will be completely healed.*

Despite the fact that they were still able to receive intravenous pain medication, the group that received the VR had pain scores that went up. The group that received VR with hypnosis had pain scores that went down. This was true both one hour and eight hours after the 40-minute VR with hypnosis treatment. Thus, the positivity and pain relief were long lasting.[30] A pain treatment that's effective in treating acute pain for eight hours without the risk of addiction! This kind of virtual reality–enhanced hypnosis has also helped burn survivors cut their use of pain medication in half.[31]

I like VR and have used it to treat patients with phobias. An inexpensive way to try this is to allow your eyes to drift open during SVT and get lost in a snowy YouTube video if you'd like to feel some cool comfort applied to burning joints—or just visualize the same thing with your mind's eye. If you really want to leave the pain in a more profound way, I recommend AVE-enhanced SVT as discussed in Chapter 6. The soothing light and sound can provide an experience that I would describe as magical and almost psychedelic in nature. If you are lying in a hospital bed covered in burns, the AVE transports you deep into the subconscious so you can create any image you'd like in your mind's eye. And the deeper the subconscious activation, the more the positivity I plant sticks.

Perhaps all these reasons are why the subconscious brain has been proven in so many studies to help with so many pain syndromes—from bad backs to somatic symptom disorder. Hypnosis helped 47 percent of subjects with chronic pain experience a "meaningful" reduction in pain, and the same reduction in pain was measured during a three-month follow-up.[32] That same researcher did a follow-up study, which revealed that only 3 percent reported "no benefit" from hypnosis. And the subjects reported that—in addition to decreased pain—they perceived increased control over pain, increased sense of relaxation and well-being, and decreased perceived stress.[33] When the researcher, continuing his line of research, asked subjects with chronic pain about short term relief of pain, hypnosis was the star. In addition to 47 percent reporting "meaningful" average reduction as cited above, 87 percent of subjects with chronic pain who received hypnosis reported a significant *immediate* reduction in pain. And the pain relief often lasts for hours.[34]

Are you beginning to see how SVT can be your brain's inner dose of prescription-strength pain relief? This also would improve your mood, which would change your perception of pain (which you may soon be able to reframe as pressure). SVT can also provide you with that "button" on your dominant finger, your own personal morphine drip to access at any time. Whenever you use this virtual PCA pump, you can bring back this inner pharmacy of pain-relieving drugs, pairing it with a deep memory of a calming experience. In just a few moments, you can experience the power of SVT to transform your pain.

WHEN A CONDITION IS MORE ELUSIVE . . .

SVT is wonderful at treating several other conditions. Since they aren't primarily autoimmune or pain syndromes, I'll call this category "elusive conditions." Make no mistake, though, the immune system is still involved, and pain is present. Irritable bowel syndrome (IBS), heartburn, migraines, overactive bladder, restless legs, leaky gut, leaky brain, small intestinal bacterial overgrowth (SIBO)—and the list goes on. Painful bladder syndrome is also in this category since it's usually more closely tied to anxiety, food sensitivities, and/or trauma. I also group colitis and Crohn's (technically autoimmune conditions) here since the way the subconscious brain addresses them is similar to the way it deals with IBS.

So, yes, this is quite a diverse set of syndromes, and they are incredibly frustrating for the people diagnosed with them. That's because modern medicine has very little to offer in the way of a treatment that actually works. And medications that do provide relief for these conditions often come at a high price in terms of side effects or risks.

As with all the other syndromes we've touched on, relevant genes can get switched on or off by your environment, which includes stress, food, or viruses. And you may have genetic "switches" that another person doesn't have: The person next to you goes through a divorce and is fine, but when you go through a stressful period, your switch for IBS gets turned on. And even IBS itself is different from one person to the next. One person develops diarrhea. The next experiences constipation. That's because the mindbody pathway is involved in all of their pathologies. These aren't rare conditions. IBS is present in 11.2 percent of adults worldwide, affecting more women than men.[35]

The subconscious brain taps into the healing process and can help with all elusive conditions on a basic level. When you activate the subconscious brain, it shifts your body from fight-or-flight mode to rest-and-digest. Too much fight-or-flight can cause, activate, or exacerbate every elusive condition I've mentioned. So the more you use SVT, the more you are putting your mindbody into rest-and-digest mode. This leads to improvements in just about every single elusive condition under the sun. After all, what condition isn't exacerbated by stress?

Hospital handouts encourage you to "manage your stress," and behavioral changes are indeed effective in helping many conditions. However, where you typically make those changes with deliberate, conscious effort, SVT helps you alleviate stress on a deeper level and make those changes in a way that becomes easy and effortless.

A moment ago, you learned how feedback loops relate to pain. Similar feedback loops, such as the gut-brain loop, are involved in elusive conditions. In gastrointestinal syndromes, your central nervous system (the brain and spinal cord) is in a two-way communication with the enteric nervous system (the one that resides in your gut). Your brain can change the levels of fluid via the hypothalamic-pituitary–adrenal axis, yet another pathway that allows the brain to communicate with the body's glands. Studies have proven the subconscious brain is effective at treating indigestion and functional chest pain (the kind that has nothing to do with your heart) through the same mindbody feedback loops. Research shows the subconscious brain can change the incoming signal from the GI tract to the brain and the outgoing messages from the brain down to the GI tract.[36] So the subconscious brain can access a master control panel that can affect any condition that's related to digestion—or, for that matter, any elusive condition.

Would you like to turn up that fluid so that things can move more smoothly? Or perhaps things are moving too quickly, and you need to tell those fluids, cells, and organs to slow down. Of course, I've just been speaking to your conscious brain. When it comes time to access the subconscious, images, colors, and metaphors work better. One doctor who specializes in IBS has a hypnosis visual he uses to treat constipation and diarrhea. Patients picture an amusement park waterslide to "get things moving" or a magical river that is slowing down.[37] You can picture that, can't you?

Does picturing poop gliding down a waterslide sound like one of those wacky "alternative treatments" that only a hard-core yogi who spends her afternoons eating muesli in Berkeley would do? Well, what does the data say? Multiple studies have shown that the subconscious brain is far more effective than any pharmaceutical drug at treating this condition—without the risk of side effects or risks.

A randomized controlled trial published in *The American Journal of Gastroenterology* used subjects who had tried and failed to treat their symptoms with medication. Of course, trying medication with little or no results is probably a situation that anyone with an elusive condition can relate to. Subjects in group one received supportive psychotherapy, which uses conscious thought to make sense of your problems. Subjects in the second group received hypnosis to change bodily functions through mysterious, deep visualizations. It was a knockout, and the winner was the subconscious brain.[38]

Another study divided subjects with IBS or functional abdominal pain (FAP) into two groups. One group was given pharmaceutical medication; the second group received six sessions of hypnosis. One year later, the group receiving medication saw their pain intensity scores fall from to an average of 8.0, from 14.1 pre-treatment. Not bad. But the group that received six sessions of hypnosis went from an average pain intensity of 13.5 pre-treatment all the way down to 1.3.[39] At a pain intensity score of 1.3, would you even classify that as "pain"? Or is that just normal, healthy pressure associated with digestion? Along the way, was the subconscious transforming pain into pressure as it was changing their bowels? No surprise: the authors of the study deemed hypnosis "highly superior" to medication. Maybe it's not so "woo-woo" to talk to your gut and bowels—or to see a poop amusement park slide—after all.

Now, since SVT is an integrative and holistic tool, you should keep seeing your functional medicine doctor or acupuncturist and going to your weekly meditation—whatever has been helping you with that elusive condition. Let's say that an at-home fecal test reveals that your gut has low levels of good bacteria. Aha! No wonder you feel anxious and your digestion is so bad—good bacteria manufacture serotonin, which makes you feel peaceful, and they help you digest food. After consulting with your prescriber, you decide you don't need to pop all those antacids or prescription antidepressants that are sometimes used to treat IBS and that come with their own set of side effects and risks. Perhaps you start taking a probiotic to address the bacteria deficiency. Problem solved, right? Not so fast. If you don't change your frazzled and stressed-out life, you'll soon kill all those new good gut bacteria. SVT can actually help you "cook" those good guys so they can multiply and thrive.

Are you starting to see how SVT can be one of many tools you use? The more elusive the "soufflé" is, the more "ingredients" you'll probably need to heal it. That makes sense, doesn't it?

Perhaps you have a food sensitivity. Your body doesn't do well with dairy, eggs, or gluten. You may be following a low-FODMAP diet, a proven strategy for people with IBS, but you struggle with adhering to the plan. I wonder if you'd be surprised to discover how SVT can help you to be successful with this regimen each and every day. You can see that delicious avocado, can't you? And a future, fabulous self who is free of the constipation or pain. And won't it be wonderful that the changes feel so easy and effortless?

Or maybe you notice that your overactive bladder or painful bladder syndrome just can't tolerate caffeine, alcohol, or artificial sweeteners at all. You may have been born with a bladder that has a very thin wall lining, or perhaps your bladder problem is related to anxiety or intimacy. Have you been to your ob-gyn, urologist, or therapist for vaginal spasms, pelvic pain, or orgasm concerns? If they've ruled out other physical disease and you have no history of abuse, it's so nice to know that your subconscious brain can help you see your future self enjoying physical intimacy, perhaps for the first time. Just as with the feedback loop between the brain and the gut, your brain can talk to your bladder and all the muscles involved in sexual function—even when you're asleep. In fact, it's just as effective in helping bed-wetting children wake up with dry sheets. In one study, children who wet the bed were either given a prescription antidepressant or received hypnosis training for three months. After six months, both groups did roughly the same: 76 percent dry beds for the antidepressant group versus 72 percent for the hypnosis group. After nine months, just 24 percent of the antidepressant group had dry beds versus 68 percent of the hypnosis group.[40]

It's pretty incredible to think that the subconscious brain—which you access during the day—can affect a physiological response that's happening while you're sleeping. Whether waking up dry or freeing yourself from bladder-related pain is a concern for you, the subconscious can speak to parts of you that the conscious brain has no control over. After all, don't all elusive conditions have an organ or function that we'd like to subconsciously turn up, down, or change in some way? Painful bladder syndrome affects about one million Americans, with about 9 in 10 of them being women; overactive bladder is even more common, affecting 17 percent of women in the U.S.[41] For the majority of patients with painful bladder syndrome who received hypnosis or listened to a guided imagery CD designed to communicate visually with the bladder, they experienced less pain,[42] less urinary urgency[43]—a symptom shared by people who struggle with painful bladder

Don't all elusive conditions have an organ or function that we'd like to subconsciously turn up, down, or change in some way?

syndrome and those who struggle with overactive bladder—and a larger improvement in overactive bladder symptoms.[44]

While we're "down there," the power of suggestion is also potent when it comes to sexual function. A British study compared testosterone, a prescription antidepressant, and hypnosis for men struggling with sexual function. Hypnosis may be your own inner "little blue pill" because it outperformed all other groups.[45]

Other studies have found the subconscious brain:

- Outperforms medication in subjects with indigestion[46]

- Changes gastric emptying and, thus, may be effective in treating gastroesophageal reflux disease (GERD)[47]

- Increases remission in subjects with ulcerative colitis[48]

- Provides relief in subjects living with cystic fibrosis[49]

You see, the subconscious can integrate the strategies you know work. We all have the resources within ourselves, and that's what your subconscious brain taps into. So whether you want to change the foods you choose to eat, communicate via the gut–brain axis, or even talk to the bladder as you sleep, harness the power of your subconscious brain to do it all.

SVT FOR BODILY HEALING

The nature of chronic pain, autoimmune diseases, and elusive conditions often develops over time—sometimes decades. These conditions have often been created by multiple factors, like a slow-cooked stew with 20 or even 30 ingredients. By the same token, your recipe for healing will also likely need time to simmer. And you may need more than just one ingredient; SVT is an integrative strategy that supports lifestyle changes or existing strategies you may use. Keep cooking this recipe of healing. With consistent use over time, this SVT practice will help reprogram your mindbody pathways. As research has shown, more use is associated with bigger boosts in immunity, pain relief, and the treatment of elusive conditions.

So let's put the seven steps of SVT to work again. This time, they'll help you improve *physical* health. SVT is potent mindbody medicine. You'll do step 1 again now as a stand-alone practice as it specifically relates to disease and discomfort. Then, steps 2 through 7 are done as one seamless practice—as you notice the body responding to the images that the subconscious brain paints.

- Step 1: Considering the Conscious

- Step 2: Activating the Subconscious

- Step 3: Revising the Past

- Step 4: Enhancing the Present

- Step 5: Creating the Future

- Step 6: Planting Positivity

- Step 7: Building Bridges

STEP 1: CONSIDERING THE CONSCIOUS

Consider those three pitfall thought patterns you wrote down on page 47. Is there one pitfall thought pattern in particular that relates to disease, physical discomfort, or dips in your physical health? Is it a thought pattern that keeps you trapped in the feedback loops of chronic pain? If it's an elusive condition, are anxious thought patterns interfering with healthy gut–brain communication . . . or communication between the brain and another organ? Does this lead to isolation—which makes you feel like this disease has become your whole life and which, of course, will depress your immune system even more? Or perhaps pain prevents you from going on the power walks you used to take around the block, which makes pain worse over the long term.

Perhaps when you review the seven pitfall thought patterns on page 44, you'll see a new pitfall thought pattern that is related to immunity, pain, or an elusive condition you wish to help. Of these seven pitfall thought patterns, here are a few that may be relevant to your concerns: If you have been diagnosed with an autoimmune condition or cancer, you may have experienced pessimism in the form of catastrophic, worst-case-scenario thinking. As you know, there's a feedback loop between mood and pain, meaning that pessimistic thought can make pain worse. If chronic pain from fibromyalgia or a car accident has been persisting for a long time, it's common to hear the pitfall thought pattern permanence as "I'm never going to feel any better." Or perhaps an elusive condition has you blaming yourself with a dose of personalization: "What's wrong with me?" Now you know that genes can get switched on by a virus or stress. It's not your fault. You may have genetic switches that other people don't, and you can do so many things to heal yourself—especially now that you have the power of your subconscious brain in your arsenal. Write the pitfall thought pattern that is specifically related to your condition here:

Type of pitfall thought pattern: _____

which, to me, is a thought that sounds something like: _____

Now that your conscious brain knows what it needs to change, your powerful subconscious brain will change it. When it comes to healing the body, some of this alchemy happens as the body begins to respond. As your digestion improves, the pitfall thought patterns vanish. You rediscover hope when you feel that moment of pain-free comfort that you hadn't felt in such a long time. Won't this be so nice to rediscover?

Find a comfortable, seated position. SVT is wonderful to use in the evening, since you can drift off to sleep afterward if you'd like. (As always, skip the optional re-alert if you're drifting off to sleep.) However, people who experience midday migraines may want to use this SVT practice during the day. Find the time that's right for you and your mindbody. Of course, be sure to re-alert yourself if you're not going to sleep right after you practice SVT. I've included this written SVT script for you to come back to when you become advanced so you can practice without the guided audio tracks. It's also a blueprint for practitioners training in SVT.

STEPS 2 THROUGH 7 OF SVT FOR BODILY HEALING

In a comfortable seated or lying posture, listen to audio track "SVT for Bodily Healing" (see page 242 for download information).

I invite you to begin this practice by allowing the eyes to close as you settle in here. And as you settle here into this comfortable state of deep relaxation, I wonder if you can bring your attention to the place in the body where you feel the most comfortable.

You already know how to activate the subconscious brain . . . and in just a moment, we'll walk through it again. I invite you to begin this journey simply . . . with a bit of mindfulness . . . by simply noticing what's on your mind—right here and right now.

And if the thoughts or feelings are related to physical sensations or your distance from ease or a syndrome that's elusive, I wonder if you can bring some gentle awareness to this space. Just notice everything you encounter here . . . imagining yourself as a magnificent and unmoving mountain. Visualizing any physical sensations that you are experiencing in this present moment—and the feelings you may have about them—as rain clouds or storms. But try as they may, they can't destroy that mountain, can they? You—that mountain—are magnificent, unmoving. You've done so much in your life—and in terms of taking care of yourself, you've done so much already to get where you are today. The fact that you're here using this practice is evidence of how much you're already taking care of yourself, isn't it?

And we all know what happens after storms, don't we? I wonder when you'll notice the most serene, still, and sunny day shining upon you. Perhaps in this present moment, it just feels so good to give yourself this time . . . with nothing to bother you . . .

nothing to do . . . except to give yourself this space to heal. After all, our body's own natural state is in the direction of healing, isn't it? You prick your finger. Your body has always known how to form a scab, hasn't it? Perhaps we can allow the excess worry that blocks this preferred healing energy to pass now—rolling on by like that one cloud blocking the sun. Like a storm cloud passing. Can you see it? Yes, your brain and body can optimize this healing energy . . . making its own Band-Aids, and in just a moment . . . we'll help that process work even better.

So now I invite you to pivot your attention to the sense of hearing. Now inviting the ears to sense **three sounds** you're hearing right here and right now. That's right. It could be interesting to begin with the loudest sound you can perceive in this moment. And now find a noise that's neither loud nor soft—a medium sound. Now, I wonder what's the quietest sound you can hear. . . . Can you hear your breath? That's right. Perfect.

And now inviting the eyes to notice two colors you can see on the back of the eyelids. The first being directly in front of you . . . and then, on the next inhale, notice a color you can see near the crown of the head as you roll the eyes up, up, up.

Now, on the next exhale . . . allow the eyes to float down, down, down . . . and then just allow the eyes to rest as any lingering tightness just floats away. Yes . . . that's right. And now I invite you to really feel this **one breath**. Allowing any tightness to give way to relaxation. Yes . . . that's right. Can you feel where the breath feels the most cool and comfortable?

In just a moment—but not quite yet—I'll invite you to use the power of your mind's eye to walk down into a healing temple of wellness. You'll see yourself step down into 12 rooms joined by a descending staircase—with each one feeling more peaceful and calm than the one you were in before. And the more calm you feel, the more you're optimizing potential for healing. Can you see the first room in front of you?

That's right. What color is the door? Is it blue-gray, or is it a soft yellow? Is there a pleasant smell of lavender . . . or is that jasmine? Perhaps you already have a sense that this journey will be a healing one.

See and feel yourself opening that first door and stepping down into the first room.

12. *Beginning to feel a pleasant sense of healing relaxation washing over you. That's right.*

11. *As you feel yourself stepping down into the next room, you'll become twice as calm as you were in the room before.*

10. *Simply allowing the mind and body to take all the time it needs. Perfect.*

9. *I wonder if you can actually feel a sense of the physical body moving down—and when you do, your bodily tension gives way to ease.*

8. *Stepping down through another doorway. That's right.*

7. *Feeling so free and comfortable now. It's almost as if every room you descend into helps you become two or even three times more relaxed than you were in the room before. And when that happens, I wonder if you'll just notice how nice this feels. Perfect.*

6. *Halfway down now. That's right. Letting go a bit more now. Isn't that such a nice feeling? Allowing your mindbody to have this time to heal. Nothing to bother you, nothing to do.*

5. *Almost there, as you step down into the next room. Isn't it so nice to know that you've already tapped into this feedback loop of healing?*

4. *Stepping down into the next room. You may notice a pleasant, dreamlike state come to you—now or at some point*

in this journey. Isn't it wonderful to know that any sort of dreamy feeling you notice means the mindbody is already at work?

3. Almost there now. That's right. You're doing so wonderfully already . . . and the healing has just begun.

2. Next-to-last room. Perfect. Feeling twice or maybe even three times as comfortable, calm, and carefree as you were on the floor before.

1. Notice now, where in your body do you feel the most relaxed? Is there a part of the body that feels particularly comfortable? If you'd like, allow that relaxation to spread over the rest of you—visualizing yourself moving it over the organ, cells, or system you'd like to optimize. Take all the time you'd like here to enjoy this type of experience you're feeling now. That's right. Good.

Now that you've felt the **body** make its way down through these rooms into this healing temple or spa you've pictured for yourself, you've probably noticed the **brain** begin to slow itself down into a calm state of healing, which, as you know, is enhancing the two-way feedback loop of healing.

In just a moment, you'll feel the body start to float upward as your consciousness begins to expand and I count up from one to seven. As these two things happen—body floating and consciousness expanding—you may notice an even deeper sense of carefree comfort and calmness. And many people notice how nice it feels when the body floats. I wonder if you'll notice that it begins to transform sensations.

As the body floats, many people also notice it feels warm—as if you're taking a warm bath or you're floating in the ocean on a spring day. Or perhaps it's as if you're falling into a cloud, and that cloud is surrounding you like a blanket. As you practice *this more, you may even find that you lose a sense of time and space. You may even find that—if you'd like—you can create a sense of "leaving" the physical body for this healing time you've given yourself. If that feels comfortable for you, you may wish to see your consciousness actually leaving the physical body as a momentary kind of "out-of-body" experience. If you'd like, for the purposes of this visualization, you can see your conscious-ness moving upward toward the sky and leaving the physical body as it floats up like a cloud. Your consciousness will return— ever so easily—to your physical body by the end of this practice or at any point during it.*

Counting now:

1. *Body floating . . . becoming as light as a feather.*

2. *Consciousness moving upward and expanding so that it's now larger than the body.*

3. *Body becoming lighter and warmer.*

4. *Consciousness moving upward and expanding even more so that it fills the room.*

5. *Body becoming almost weightless now.*

6. *Consciousness moving so elevated and expanded that it's like a cloud in the sky.*

7. *So deep and so relaxed. Perfect.*

In just a moment, but not quite yet, I'll invite the subconscious to help you here. For the purposes of this practice, I'll invite your subconscious to light up positive, pain-free, and pleasurable memories from your past—by doing this, it will help re-create those same pathways for you right here and right now. So in just a moment, you'll float back in time with the power of your subconscious brain . . . going back to a time when you felt truly content . . . truly comfortable . . . truly carefree. I don't know if that time was yesterday or 20 years ago, and that really doesn't matter. What matters is that you call upon the unique power of your subconscious brain to fully re-create this feeling as best you can. As you know, the subconscious is so adept at re-creating visual and visceral memories.

Pressing play on that positive, pain-free, and pleasurable scene from your past and inviting the eyes to slowly flutter side to side a bit now on three . . . two . . . one . . . [left-right-left-right audio tones].

Now, inhale on the count of three: one, two, three. Exhale on the count of six: one, two, three, four, five, six. What did you see? Imagine that the next breath you take is bathing your cells in the feeling of that energy. What does it feel like? You can feel that, can't you?

I wonder whether the subconscious, if only for the briefest moment, has helped you tap into your own inner pharmacy of endorphins and anti-inflammatory agents by helping you to feel just one percent more free or comfortable . . . or was it even more than one percent? Either way, you have just discovered how to tap into your own inner morphine or anti-inflammatory agent or immune-booster drip—one that's natural and risk-free. Isn't that wonderful? Most people continue to feel more and more comfortable every time they use this practice. . . . Does that bring you a sense or comfort . . . or is it control? If only for this moment, remind the brain and the body what this feels like. Try this on again. You never really forget how to ride a bike once you've learned, do you? Or how to swim . . . although you also probably aren't as good at riding a bike or as good at swimming if you haven't done it in a long time, are you? So now let's remind that mindbody feedback loop that, as you know, it is a two way communication from brain to body and body to brain . . . so that all the cells and organs know what to look for—this comfort and carefree ease you feel now—and *show them what they should create . . . since ease, comfort, and healing is actually your innate and natural state. If you have found just one memory in your past where you felt comfortable and carefree, then you already have the muscle memory for this pathway. Now remind every one of your cells that you know how to be free.*

So review that positive, pain-free, and pleasurable scene one more time. And this time, I wonder if you can optimize healing even more. Can you really remind brain and body what it feels like and turn up your inner immune infantry or pain-free bliss just a bit more? By changing your awareness, you can enhance the potential for healing. Or, if you'd like, you could simply crank the dial for healing up as high as it goes. Make it feel even better than it did the time before. Pressing play, invite the eyes to slowly flutter now on three . . . two . . . one . . . [left-right-left-right audio tones].

Now inhale on the count of three: one, two, three. Exhale on the count of six: one, two, three, four, five, six. Did you feel it? Allowing yourself to just spread that around . . . every organ. All that healing energy. Seeing it, sensing it . . . so serene now. That's right. Perfect.

And now, moving forward, visualizing yourself in present day . . . which organ or system would you like to optimize or heal? You've probably realized that you have inner abilities to heal yourself, haven't you? Now visualize all those abilities gathering in your dominant hand. If you'd like, take the dominant hand and place it over the system you're healing today . . . or if you'd prefer and it's more comfortable for you, simply visualize that happening in your mind's eye. That's right . . . and you've already cultivated so much carefree comfort. I wonder if you can gather all the healing potential you've already noticed here today—whether it was in the brain or in the body—and visualize that energy coming out of your hand. I don't know if the energy will look like a cool blue wave or a warm red pulse

. . . and it really doesn't matter, because your own subconscious brain knows exactly what kind of energy you need. Release your own inner heating pad or make it feel like Icy Hot . . . like a cool menthol. If the hand is on your head, perhaps it's bringing a sense of relief . . . or just slowing the brain down. That's right. Many people will notice, as they visualize this, an inner reminder: My own mindbody knows how to heal itself. Nothing to bother me, nothing to do; I'm in control of my own comfort. And now, placing the hand back in a resting position or visualizing it returning ever so gently . . . know that this hand is now uniquely ordained to heal whenever you need it. In the future, placing the hand on any area—while practicing SVT or in your waking, everyday life—this will act as a reminder for your subconscious brain to unlock the mindbody healing potential.

Now I invite you to access the master control panel of your own inner healing system. Can you see that control panel? I wonder if it looks like the cockpit of an old 747 plane with manual controls and levers or if it's more like a modern one that's controlled by an iPad. You can see it, can't you? Now, I imagine you already have an idea of what needs to change. Can you see that dial for immunity? Would you like to turn up that dial? Or perhaps you'd like to access your detoxification pathways. Or both? And how about those sensation pathways that can transform pain into pressure? I wonder if you'd like to hack into that panel—and visualize the subconscious brain turning it down, down . . . all the way down. That's right. And now turn up the dial that notices pleasant sensations. That's interesting. The pathways are becoming totally scrambled, aren't they? Pleasantness trumps pain, and pain becomes pressure, and you've just pulled the trigger that turns on this healing pathway. And since comfort begets more comfort, you've just created an upward spiral . . . doesn't that just soothe you or cheer you? Or is it the esophagus, gut, or bladder that needs adjusting? As you already know, the subconscious has access to all these bodily functions—so go ahead and tweak any levers and dials that you'd like. And as you do, I wonder where you'll notice a change. Some people notice a calmness in the brain, others a comfort in the body, and still others something beginning to change in that pathway between the two. That's right. Perfect.

And now imagine you have a special sort of healing light—one that looks like a scan or a laser. It's going to pass over every part of the body, from the head to the toe, which will seal and optimize all the healing that's already taken place. This special laser can do anything at all, and you may wish to visualize anything it touches transforming. As it touches that tension headache, does it transform into a ball that you can move, shrink, and change? Moving to the shoulders now, transforming that tension from red . . . now pink . . . now blue . . . now soft white . . . can you feel it? As the light and energy and color you see in your mind's eye makes contact with each organ and cell, it may feel cool and comfortable in areas that feel warm. In the gut, can you feel the ease? Your immune system can be quite colorful—see it moving to the places you need extra healing, and see the color changing as it also helps the healthy cells. Is this special laser-like scan helping things to move more regularly and quickly, or for you, is it more slowly? It may act as an anti-inflammatory or talk to any organs—speeding them up or slowing them down in any way. Moving down now to the bladder, the genitals . . . all the way down to the feet . . . scanning through the mindbody. One connected entity, working with you—not against you. Just noticing these advanced feedback loops and advanced connections that have always been here . . . conspiring in your favor.

Now move that healing scan up and down the body—and visualize your subconscious brain doing anything at all it still needs to do. Continuing to tinker with all sorts of outgoing and incoming messages along feedback loops. This healing laser is locking in the reprogramming among your brain, your body, and the complex pathways that allow communication and con-

nection between cells. From now on, anything not serving you may disappear, and sensations may change. And you'll notice pleasant sensations more than ever before. And all this comfort will begin to beget more comfort.

With this image, know that you have already begun to heal. I don't know if you'll feel the effects right away or if you'll feel them as they multiply over time—and that doesn't matter, because you're already here on this healing journey. And wherever you are, the longest journey starts with a single step . . . and since you're hearing these words, your trip has already begun.

Now allow the subconscious brain to paint this all step-by-step—whatever it is that needs to unfold from start to finish. Since all healing processes can be optimized with food, see healing foods on your plate. And see it as an energy; perhaps you could see it as pure love—after all, weren't there people who gave their time and energy away from their families to harvest that berry so that you could have that food? And that food is going to nourish your body . . . to help you heal, isn't it? Then, perhaps you can see all the incredible processes in your brain and body—from salivation to passage through the intestines—that helps you break down that food into energy and, of course, reap the benefits of all of the antioxidants that keep your cells healthy. And they help detoxify the body, keep the immune system strong, and prevent inflammation, keeping the body in a state of comfort and ease. . . . See it passing through you at just the right speed at just the right time . . . with a state of gratitude. Isn't it so nice that everything—from exercise to food to sleep to relationships—is all there to nourish you? And the more we use these natural, holistic strategies, the more the brain and the body are healthy and whole. Whatever your journey may be, see the process unfold in healing energies from start to finish. Isn't it interesting that every food, every doctor, and every family member has already been a part of your journey?

Now fast-forward to a time in the future. In just a moment, you'll see the future version of yourself—the one who is fabulous and flourishing, carefree and confident. What are you seeing in the future? It's happening right now. . . . What are you feeling now? Can you see that picture now? What do you look like . . . so happy, so healthy and so pain-free? What are you doing now . . . right now? What do you smell? What are you eating? That's right. Really painting that picture now. Fully embodying your future self . . . as you allow this to wash over your entire being, reprogramming brain and body, and the feedback loop that travels between them, to look out for this version of you. Here you are, in this present moment, feeling so free.

Also see anything you need to do—and the small, everyday steps that will allow you to get there. From using this practice again to the foods you eat to treatments you're already using, they will all have a synergistic effect to help you create this future. Allow these next few minutes to seem much longer . . . so you can see it all unfolding step-by-step and day by day . . . in an easy and effortless way. And when you feel any sense of these sensations, you'll be reminding brain and body what they need to look for. That's right. That's right. You're doing just fine.

In just a moment, I'll have you float even deeper one more time—so that we can plant the seeds of positivity and healing deep into the subconscious. Now deepening this wonderful feeling of being so carefree and comfortable as I count down from three to one: three . . . two . . . one . . . that's right. I wonder if you'll notice a sense of relaxation in a part of your body or if you feel a bit better in the way you think. Either way, it's so nice to know that you have control . . . because whether you've made a tiny change or a profound one, you created that, didn't you? And these changes are just the beginning—especially when it comes to complex bodily processes, immune optimization, and healing. I'm not sure if you'll notice a part of your body feeling better tomorrow when you wake up or if you'll slowly notice digestion or another organ working better in a few weeks. You have already begun to heal. Because you've practiced this technique here today, you have already affected positive change. Isn't it so nice to know that you've already set this domino effect into motion? And you'll encounter a situation—whether it's a food or an activity—where you'll notice that a pathway begins to feel a bit different. I'm not sure when that will be for you, but when you do, you'll realize that you've already begun to reprogram the mindbody. This will make you want to return to this practice so you can reprogram it a bit more. And this carefree comfort will continue to grow like a snowball—during your waking hours and even while you sleep—because by practicing this today, you've helped return your body to its natural state: one of healing.

Now it's time to build a bridge—so you can take everything you've gained from this healing practice into your future for continued optimal health. Whenever you need to be reminded of anything and everything you have discovered here, you'll have a way to do so. The first part of building this bridge involves a button.

First, I want you to find the three best things you've gained here. Perhaps they were sensations or pathways that you hadn't felt activated in a long time. It could be a direct healing pathway to any organ you'd like. Or were they feelings or reminders? You could visualize this as pure healing energy if you'd like—I wonder what color that would be. Now send the best part of this healing energy down your dominant arm into your dominant hand. Gather and intensify this feeling of comfort or activation in your dominant index finger. If you'd like, it could be your own button for the most powerful anti-inflammatory, pain-relieving, immune-boosting medication the world has ever known. That's right. Now rub the tip of that index finger with that thumb. Can you feel that? Just there. You've just built a button for yourself. Whenever you need a little piece of what you've created here, all you need to do is to push that button. All the healing or comfort will come flooding back. You can use this button on its own, and it will even help other integrative strategies work better too. Isn't it so nice to know this button is here . . . to realign you with your own natural state: healing and carefree comfort? That's right.

Second, gather any residual discomfort you'd like to get rid of right now—any leftover tension or nausea or pain . . . or feelings about those sensations. Now I invite you to visualize that a balloon is tied to your nondominant index finger. Can you feel it? See that balloon being blown up as you fill it with the "hot air" of the energy that blocks your natural healing state. Many people may even notice that the finger begins to lift a bit here on its own. Isn't that interesting? Just one last moment here—see if there's one last ounce of pessimism or pain you'd like to send into that balloon. That's right. And now rub that thumb against your nondominant index finger—which will untie the balloon from the finger. In your mind's eye, see that balloon float far, far away . . . and perhaps you'll even feel that finger floating back down. Can you see the balloon becoming so small? Tiny now? Follow it until it's gone. And in the future, whenever you need to free yourself from tension or discomfort, all you need to do is put those sensations into this balloon that's tied to your nondominant index finger. Then, rub your thumb to untie the string . . . and let it all go. In each and every moment, you have the power to set yourself free. As you get better and better . . . in each moment . . . every moment . . . taking this healing journey day by day.

OPTIONAL RE-ALERT

And now see yourself walking back up—through the rooms you walked through to get here. Stepping up into each room in ascending order. Becoming twice as alert and awake and returning back to your everyday, waking state. You'll feel your consciousness returning to your body so effortlessly. That's right.

1. *Feeling yourself becoming alert now.*

2. *As you ascend, becoming more awake . . . and even hopeful for tomorrow.*

3. *Perhaps give a wiggle to your fingers and your toes. Feel this incredible body of yours, and as you do, feel more and more awake.*

4. *That's right. Up and activated.*

5. *Twice as energized and alert as the step before.*

6. *Stepping up again.*

7. *Really feeling all the energy return to your mind and body.*

8. *That's right.*

9. *Alert and activated . . . and wiggling those fingers and toes a bit more in this carefree body now.*

10. *Feeling your body ascend.*

11. *Almost there.*

12. *Eyes open. And when they do, feeling hopeful for the healing and the life that is yours.*

To ensure you're fully conscious again, look around the room and name aloud 10 items you see, take a walk around the block, listen to some upbeat music, or do 25 jumping jacks.

APPENDIX A

Bonus SVT Practice for Sleep, Insomnia, and Induced Dreaming

Insomnia impacts your biological rhythms, your focus, and your relationships—and not in a good way. If you struggle with sleeplessness, then you already know the toll it can take. So wouldn't it be nice if you were able to put your insomnia to bed and keep it there? SVT is a powerful way to help you drift into an easy slumber and rest more deeply.

When you're falling asleep, your brain slows down—from the fast brain waves of everyday life into the slower theta and delta brain waves (dreaming and dreamless sleep, respectively). When you're sleeping, these brain waves fluctuate. Recent research has demonstrated that sleep and dreaming may be even more vital to our health than we could imagine. The longer you stay asleep, the more frequently your brain surfaces from delta to theta brain waves. These brain waves can even act as a replacement for night-time dreaming.

In my book *The Brain Fog Fix*, I wrote about why sufficient sleep is vital: "A 2013 animal study showed that during sleep, channels between neurons expand up to 60 percent, which allows cerebrospinal fluid in. All that extra space between neurons is your brain getting ready to get hosed down: the cerebrospinal fluid flushes out the Alzheimer's disease–causing plaques. This 'wash cycle' is much more effective when you're asleep, which means more 'junk' gets cleared from your brain.[1]

"That's why it came as no surprise when another study found that mice who sleep for only four hours a day had more Alzheimer's-causing plaques in the brain.[2] Sleep might also reinforce brain cells; a 2013 study showed that while mice slept, their brains were making more myelin, the brain cells' insulation that allows the electrical current of happiness to flow freely.[3]"

Fortunately, there are several ways to improve sleep, and they involve both parts of your brain.

CONSCIOUS BRAIN FOR BETTER SLEEP

The conscious brain is pretty good at improving sleep. In *Heal Your Drained Brain*, I created a unique, three-level version of cognitive behavioral therapy for insomnia (CBT-I). CBT-I is a natural way to treat insomnia. In 2016, the American College of Physicians recommended CBT-I as the initial treatment—rather than medication—for adults with insomnia.[4] This group is the largest medical-specialty organization in the United States, so this is an important decree for health professionals and patients alike. They're encouraging CBT-I while trying to reverse the overprescribing and overconsumption of sleeping pills that has occurred in the past decade.

Level 1 of CBT-I uses some basic sleep hygiene tips, such as dimming the lights before bed and learning to associate your bed with being asleep. Levels 2 and 3 use exercises, poses, and mathematical equations. Level 3 helps you "compress" your sleep and then "expand" it, initially forcing you to sleep less so that you can become naturally tired. CBT-I is basically a scientific and natural way to realign your natural sleep-wake cycles. See Chapter 12 in *Heal Your Drained Brain* for more details and the full, three-level CBT-I program.

SUBCONSCIOUS BRAIN FOR BETTER SLEEP

Yes, it's vital to sleep about eight hours. But it's not just about sleep itself. You see, dreams aren't just noise and nonsense. Mainstream, modern science is beginning to realize that dreams, their associated rapid eye movement (REM), and the theta brain wave state are vital for brain health—and not just psychological or spiritual but also physical well-being. Research in 2017 associated a lack of REM sleep with both depression and dementia. As the researcher who authored this study observed, "Everything we see, every conversation we have, is chewed on and swallowed and filtered through while we dream, and either excreted or assimilated."[5]

As you already know, SVT is incredible for helping you do all those things that researcher mentioned: chew on, swallow, filter, excrete, and assimilate your memories, thoughts, and desires. Unlike dreams that occur during sleep, the dreamy scenes you can create with SVT are in your control. What would you like to chew on and swallow? Which thoughts do you want to filter through a more positive lens? I wonder what scenes you'll choose to excrete so you get better rest.

Since theta brain waves have been shown to make people feel drowsy and fall asleep,[6] SVT can also help you spend more time sleeping—and that means more dreaming. Since the vast majority of theta-dominant dreaming occurs during the fifth and final phase of your sleep cycle, you miss out on the healing power of dreams and REM if you are only sleeping six hours. In fact, dreaming may act as a preventative tonic against developing PTSD. Research has found that people who spend more time in REM have less fear the next day when under conditions that mimic stress or trauma.[7] Thus, you want to sleep a good, solid eight hours to have spontaneously occurring dreams and use SVT to supplement nighttime dreaming with at-will dreams.

SVT can also improve sleep quality by boosting slow-wave sleep. A groundbreaking 2014 study used a quick subconscious brain–activating audio track and then measured the subjects' sleep quality with an EEG. Subjects got deeper, more restful sleep thanks to the activation of the subconscious brain.[8]

A COMBO APPROACH

To help with sleep issues, you can use SVT as detailed elsewhere in this book. In step 1, you would examine the pitfall thought pattern that is preventing deep and restful sleep. It may be helpful to examine the past and visualize yourself falling asleep effortlessly and easily in your future. But you could also supercharge this process by adding the level of CBT-I that fits your particular sleep issues. Then, while you're visiting your past, present, and future in SVT, see yourself using the CBT-I strategies through the week. Won't it be so nice to see yourself effortlessly implementing CBT-I techniques and sleeping soundly?

In a comfortable position in bed, listen to the audio track "SVT for Sleep, Insomnia & Induced Dreaming" (see page 242 for download information) to help you fall asleep and stay asleep.

SVT FOR SLEEP, INSOMNIA & INDUCED DREAMING

The following brief bonus SVT track will help you to fall asleep and sleep more deeply. This script has elements of subconscious brain–activation to increase slow-wave sleep,[9] mindfulness meditation, and guided visualization.

Begin by lying down in your bed and getting comfortable.

Center and relax yourself by becoming mindful of your senses. I wonder what five things you see right here and right now. That's right. How about finding four sounds? Now I wonder what three sensations you can notice . . . brought to you courtesy of your skin. Are there two scents lingering? And I wonder if you could even find one thing you can taste—something lingering on the tongue . . . that peppermint tea, perhaps? Isn't it so nice to know that your senses are always here to help you become so still in any moment you'd like?

Now, would you like to become even more relaxed? I invite you to take one hand and place it about a foot or so in front of the face with the elbow slightly bent and with all five fingers touching. That's right. Now fix your gaze on the middle finger . . . becoming more and more relaxed. You don't even have to focus the eyes . . . it will be as if you're looking past the middle finger.

When the hand appears to be going a bit out of focus, that will be an indication that your body has become even more deeply relaxed here . . . with nothing to bother you and nothing to do. Isn't it so nice to have this time to relax . . . so you can rest and restore yourself? And now I wonder at what point your subconscious will become activated. It may be in just a moment—and it may happen quite quickly. Or you may notice it happening slowly throughout this practice. As you already know, when your subconscious takes over, it simply means you are relaxing in a deep way.

Simply notice where you feel the relaxation the most right now. You can feel that, can't you? When you notice it, then one or more of the fingers will begin to spread. I don't know which finger will move first . . . will it be the index finger? Or will it be the thumb? Or perhaps all five fingers will spread at the same time.

When that first finger moves, you'll also notice that the hand and the arm become a bit limp. I wonder if it even begins to feel a bit heavy . . . or even hard to hold it up. That's right. So as you let go, just allow gravity to move the hand closer and closer to the face. Closer and closer. Deeper and deeper. Nothing to bother you; nothing to do.

Whenever the hand touches some part of your face, allow the eyelids to close. And find a comfortable place to rest the hand . . . that's right. Perfect.

As the eyelids close, a feeling of restorative rest will begin to wash over you . . . easing the mind and relaxing the body. On the next inhale of the lungs, gently roll the eyes up a bit if you'd like. And then, on the next exhale, allow the eyes to roll back down to neutral . . . allowing yourself to release into an even deeper state of rejuvenating rest. That's right. Nothing to bother you . . . nothing to do.

I invite you to now imagine you're on an escalator. This escalator moves you down . . . 12 . . . 11 . . . 10 . . . twice as drowsy and relaxed on every floor . . . 9 . . . 8 . . . 7 . . . nothing to bother you and nothing to do . . . 6 . . . 5 . . . 4 . . . just allowing yourself to drift as you move down . . . 3 . . . 2 . . . 1 . . . that's right. Feeling more relaxed than you were just minutes ago. And isn't it nice that you did that for yourself? You deserve this time to rest. After all, the more you allow yourself this restorative time, the more energetic and better you'll be tomorrow. So just . . . let . . . go . . . that's right. Perfect.

Now imagine a conveyer belt in your mind's eye . . . and on this conveyer belt are any thoughts that are lingering. . . . You can simply picture any thoughts or feelings that come up in this moment moving on that conveyer belt . . . and that belt deposits any conscious thoughts or to-do-list tasks into a bottle. Can you see that bottle?

And now . . . or at any time throughout this practice . . . simply place anything you'd like into that bottle and rest in the comfort of knowing that you can look at this bottle tomorrow or the next day. As soon as you picture this bottle, you'll notice that your conscious and subconscious brain both begin to let go . . . after all, you can pick up this bottle tomorrow, can't you? And actually, the more you free yourself from these thoughts now . . . the more your brain will be able to handle them tomorrow. For now, this is your time to rest, relax, and restore your brain and body.

And now I'd like you to picture a feather. Is it a large white one? Or is it a small blue feather? You see this feather floating in the air. Perhaps you can imagine that you are that feather . . . and ever so gently and ever so easily, you're floating down on a wisp of air. As you gently float, you fall into this deeper and deeper relaxing state. If you'd like, you could even see this feather floating down to the tune of a lullaby. That's right . . .

And the more this feather simply floats down on a bed of air, the deeper your sleep will become. That's right . . . that's right . . .

Whenever you'd like to float down into this state of rest at any time in the future, all you'll need to do is to remember this feather. . . . You can also press that button on your dominant index finger . . . and your brain's inner pharmacy of soothing, sleep-promoting brain chemicals will be released. . . . You may even hear a lullaby playing softly whenever you press this button. You can also gently ask the subconscious to give you the most pleasant dreams.

In your dreams, the subconscious brain may even help you to assimilate memories . . . helping you to transfer important lessons and memories from today into long-term drawers . . . and knowing exactly which files it needs to throw out . . . and in a pleasant way, it can even show you something about yourself and your desires or your destiny in your dreams.

And then you'll float so easily down to dreamless sleep . . . I don't know exactly if you'll have a pleasant dream first or deep and dreamless sleep first . . . or dreamless sleep first and then the most peaceful and pleasant dreams . . . it doesn't really matter right now . . . because your brain knows exactly how it needs to rest . . . and dream. Cycling though this in ways it already knows how to do—without you needing to do anything. . . . Just rest. That's right. That's right.

You'll probably feel more and more like that feather . . . floating oh so gently now . . .

Nothing to bother you; nothing to do . . .

Deeper and deeper . . .

Just relaxing in this rejuvenating and restful state . . .

Deeper and deeper . . .

Floating and feeling so relaxed . . .

That's right . . .

That's right . . .

Rest.

APPENDIX B

Bonus SVT Practice for Success

Would you like to tap into the power of your subconscious brain to become even more successful? By now, you've already used SVT to delete naysaying voices. Isn't it so nice to fill your brain with inspiring ones, the ones that lift you up? I wonder if it'd be inspiring to walk into that boardroom and close a multi-million-dollar deal as though it were no big deal. Let's take that cool, calm confidence you've already cultivated and take it to the next level—specifically harnessing the power of the subconscious to make you more successful. It's an incredible skill that can help you become more confident or creative in your career.

With SVT you can transform any energy that feels like desperation to clients into *owning* your inherent self-worth. You have a unique set of skills, unique experience, and a reason to be here, don't you? Don't you wonder how tapping into this energy will help clients feel lucky to work with you? Along the way, would you like to unleash the true power of your creative potential? What brilliant idea will your subconscious brain hatch and visualize—and then see through with conviction?

Up to this point, all the SVT practices I've walked you through have been fairly long. But you can actually practice SVT for 5 or 45 minutes. My website, drmikedow.com, has several SVT practices of varying lengths for various goals and concerns. Now that you've had a chance to practice it, you've probably become skilled at activating your subconscious brain. After all, it is a skill—just like learning to play a new sport. Every time you use this practice, you'll get a bit faster.

Here, I'll offer you a bonus SVT practice for success. It's quick, so you could even use it in your car or office just before a big meeting. Repeat step 1 if you'd like (refer back to Chapter 3), particularly if you sense that a pitfall thought pattern is blocking you from success. Otherwise, you can jump right into this SVT practice for success.

In a comfortable seated posture, listen to the audio track "SVT to Boost Your Success" (see page 242 for download information) to boost your confidence and build success.

SVT FOR SUCCESS

*As you close the eyes, ground yourself right here and right now—which is really wonderful for helping you feel centered and peaceful. What are **three sounds** you're noticing? Notice **two colors** on the back of the eyelids—the first straight out in front of you . . . and on your next inhale, see a color near the crown of the head as you look up, up, up. And on the next exhale, allow the eyes to float down, down, down . . . and just find a neutral place to just rest and relax. That's right. Now just really enjoy this **one breath**. Can you feel the rib cage expanding by one millimeter or the air warming the nostrils? That's right. Perfect.*

*And now see yourself boarding an elevator with **12 floors**.*

12 . . . 11 . . . 10 . . . Ten floors down and feeling confident, cool, and calm.

9 . . . 8 . . . 7 . . . Seven floors down and feeling twice as relaxed on every floor.

6 . . . 5 . . . 4 . . . Four floors down and noticing how carefree and comfortable you are.

3 . . . 2 . . . 1 . . . That's right. . . . Stepping out onto this floor— this place that embodies true confidence . . . you can feel it, can't you? Yes . . . you already can feel your worth.

I wonder, can you turn up this inner feeling of self-worth and success? You'll feel them in the body just a bit more as I count upward from one to seven. One . . . two . . . three . . . four . . . five . . . six . . . seven . . . that's right. Perfect.

And now I want you to rewind the tape of your life to access all the incredible things you have done. All your success. All your achievements. I wonder if you can find a time in your life when you have felt so confident. Go back to that memory . . . that time. What do you see? How does it feel? It's so interesting to take a moment to remember that, yes, you've already achieved so much, haven't you? And while you're finding this confidence, also find that part of you that reminds you of your purpose . . . why you do what you do. I wonder if it's a specific memory—or is it more a general feeling? Is this your true calling? Or perhaps this is something you're doing so you can help others in a different way, serving others and your family . . . or getting this job as a stepping-stone toward your calling. Either way, you've found an inner well of passion and purpose. I wonder what it feels like to recall that. . . . That's right.

And now, fast-forwarding into your present life, allow that cool, collected sense of confidence . . . everything that you have already achieved . . . and everything that you already are . . . to wash over the present you. Remind your present self how competent and capable you already are. I wonder if it's calming you . . . or is it making you sit up a bit straighter now? Is this confidence speaking to your shoulders—as you now feel a bit taller, a bit prouder? Or is it affecting the confidence of your thoughts? Many people notice that this confidence unlocks the floodgates of creativity . . . and you may even notice a gamma wave—that "aha" moment—pop up at some point during this practice. Wherever you notice a small change—in your brain or in your body—visualize that confident, creative self . . . spreading all over you . . . visualizing it as a color if you'd like.

And now see your future unfold . . . right here and right now. I wonder if you can see yourself in a meeting that's going to happen with a client in just a few moments . . . or in just a few weeks? Or are you in a studio? Wherever you are, visualize it. What are you doing and seeing? Feel it. How does that feel? During this practice, time is floating away . . . so a few seconds can feel like an hour. So rehearse anything you need to do to cultivate success . . . to see this all unfolding step-by-step. It also helps you to remain flexible . . . because with your cool, calm confidence, you're actually prepared for anything that life throws at you, aren't you? Haven't you already achieved so much? That's right.

Deepening one more time as I count from three to one to plant positivity deep into your subconscious . . . three . . . two . . . one. . . . At some point in the future . . . which may be in just a few minutes . . . or perhaps on a call at your desk . . . or when you're on stage . . . or speaking publicly—wherever you may be, at some point you'll be surprised at how confident and calm and creative you are. I wonder where you will be when you notice that something has changed. Will it be in your mind? Or will you notice a change in your body? Many people notice the change happening in both places. Because you have already achieved so much . . . this change isn't outside of you . . . it's within you . . . and it will all unfold in a way that feels easy and effortless. And you'll stay calm and collected. After all, you've just seen and experienced everything that's about to unfold, haven't you?

Now I invite you to send this confidence to a button in your dominant index finger. So whenever you need a dose of this cool, calm, creative energy, all you need to do is press this button with your thumb. And now gather any residual self-doubt— visualizing it now as you blow it all into a balloon tied to your nondominant index finger. Now untie that balloon with your thumb . . . and watch as it floats far, far away. Can you see it becoming small?

Now board that elevator . . . and in just a moment, become more alert on every floor . . . and by the time your reach floor one, you'll be fully awake, ready to take this cool, calm, creative, and confident you into the world . . . to create this success.

12 . . . 11 . . . 10 . . . Ten floors up, becoming more alert.

9 . . . 8 . . . 7 . . . Seven floors up, wiggling your fingers and toes.

6 . . . 5 . . . 4 . . . Four floors up, conscious with confidence

3 . . . 2 . . . 1 . . . Eyes open. Awake. Alert. Cool and confident you.

APPENDIX C

Bonus SVT Practice for Spiritual Connection

As you already know, SVT is part of a holistic approach to wellness. It's a bio-psycho-social-spiritual approach. Scientifically speaking, the subconscious brain can change consciousness—affecting your perception of time and space, self-orientation, and attention. But you can also use the subconscious to deepen your spiritual practice or beliefs. It's been said that if the soul lived in a part of the brain, it'd be in the prefrontal cortex—an area of the brain that lights up when activated by the subconscious. In terms of brain waves, angels would reside in theta, which, as you know, are the signature of the subconscious.

Where do you find spiritual fulfillment and connection in your life? Do you find it in nature, in a place of worship, or both? Dreams are another potential source of spiritual connection. Most people have had a dream with some sort of deeper meaning, so you probably already understand how the subconscious can enrich this part of your life.

Of course, I'm not here to tell you what to believe. In my private practice, I treat people from all faiths while respecting their beliefs. SVT is equally open and affirming. Whatever your beliefs may be, this therapeutic partnering with the subconscious brain can enhance and deepen your spiritual practice. By becoming profoundly still via the subconscious brain, you can feel at one with the universe, all living beings, the divine, your loved ones, or a higher power. Which imagery speaks most to you? The subconscious can help you have an out-of-body experience as it changes areas in the brain associated with self-orientation, time, and space.

I wonder how SVT will help you tap into your unique set of gifts—and how you will use these to be of service. Some deep part of you knows there's something you were meant to do to fill the world with more love, doesn't it? How does tapping into something greater than yourself transform your existence?

Some people use SVT to have conversations with people they have lost, and this helps them to heal. Perhaps you believe the words you say via SVT travel to heaven, or maybe you believe this time is for you to use the power of the subconscious brain to see and hear things left unsaid. Would you like to be in communion with God or angels? Perhaps you believe that your words are traveling directly to the soul of your lost loved one, or perhaps you simply believe that the healing is happening in a part of your own brain. I imagine either scenario would be peaceful and healing for a person who is healing.

Here's an SVT practice for spiritual deepening. Find a quiet and peaceful place. You may wish to light a candle, incense, or sage—anything that helps you to deepen your spiritual practice.

In a comfortable seated or lying-down position, listen to the audio track "SVT to Deepen Your Spiritual Practice" (see page 242 for download information) to reconnect with your higher power or life purpose.

SVT FOR SPIRITUAL DEEPENING

*As you close the eyes, ground yourself in this precious moment of the right here and right now. Can you feel this beautiful earth rising up to support your body? And now gently bring your attention to **three sounds** you're noticing. And now, can you no-*

*tice **two colors** on the back of the eyelids? Notice the first one straight out in front of you . . . and on your next inhale, see a color near the crown of the head as you look up, up, up. And on the next exhale, allow the eyes to float down, down, down . . . that's right. Now just really enjoy this **one breath**. Can you feel the rib cage expanding by one millimeter or the air warming the nostrils? That's right. Perfect.*

*Now envision yourself leaning back—like you're doing a trust fall off a picnic table and falling back into a heavenly cloud. This cloud feels so supportive . . . so still . . . and so serene. And it gently lulls your soul down **12 floors**. It's almost as if this cloud is taking you away from this earthly world for a moment and toward a deeper and more spiritual existence.*

12 . . . 11 . . . 10 . . . Floating down . . . feeling so still and so calm . . .

9 . . . 8 . . . 7 . . . Drifting down now . . . with a feeling of peace and purpose . . .

6 . . . 5 . . . 4 . . . As this heavenly cloud takes you down to a place that's infinitely safe and supremely supportive . . .

3 . . . 2 . . . 1 . . . That's right . . . floating down into the most spiritual, serene, and still place you can imagine. You can see it, can't you?

And now, as I count from one to seven . . . can you enhance this feeling of spiritual connection even more? If you'd like, you can even have a brief out-of-body experience where earthly time and space float away for the brief time of this practice. Your soul will come easily back down into the body, into earthly time, at the end of this practice because you're not done here . . . you have so much important work left to do here. But even so, I'd imagine it'd be so soothing to have a glimpse. Of your spirit . . . your soul . . . the other side . . . or whatever is in line with your spiritual beliefs. Counting now. One . . . two . . . three . . . four . . . five . . . six . . . seven . . . that's right. Perfect.

And now invite the subconscious and perhaps even your soul . . . to take you back—back as far as you'd like to go. I don't know where you'll go today. Perhaps it's back to a time when you were still wide-eyed and innocent, ready to change the world. Did you forget that you still have that innocent little girl or boy inside of you? He or she is still right here . . . and can make a difference. Maybe you can imagine that you are there, watching your childhood as a spectator. Or if you believe in destiny, imagine you're there before this earthly time existed . . . before you were even born. Either way, you can now see exactly what gifts and talents you were given, can't you? I wonder how you were meant to develop these gifts to better the world. Have you forgotten how inherently worthy you are? Some part of you knows that, doesn't it? Or do you need to go back and have a conversation with someone who has passed? Perhaps you can imagine your old self having a conversation with God or a higher power or your highest self. What path would have been different? See that past unfold . . . right here and right now. Or I wonder if there is something even more spiritual in nature—that's not of this physical world. Allow your soul to find whatever that may be . . .

Now fast-forward to your present, earthly life. With the spiritual deepening you just created in your past, what is different in the present? I wonder if your present life is supercharged with just a little more spirit. What do you see? Most people see more love, more connection, more peace. How does this feel? I wonder if you'd like to even feel this as a soft-white spiritual light that is spilling out of your pores—and this light begins to touch everyone you come in contact with. What are you doing differently? From your thoughts to your words to your deeds, what has changed? I wonder how this sense of peace and purpose has changed your present life . . . and how it affects others like a rock being dropped in a lake. The ripples of your spirit touching everyone for miles . . .

And now, moving into the future . . . see the future version of yourself . . . your highest self, which is, of course a deep and profoundly evolved one . . . right here and right now. What's the best part? Is it the stillness or the serenity? Is it the peace or the purpose? If you'd like, you can even picture yourself connected to all beings—transcending the physical body or the physical world a bit more. Can you turn up that feeling? That's right. That's right. Perfect. And that's what you are . . . you beautiful creature, you. You are already perfect. I wonder how you will continue to find the beauty in yourself . . . and by realizing this, bring out the true inner beauty in others.

And deepening one more time as I count from three to one to plant positivity deep into your subconscious and your soul . . . three . . . two . . . one. . . . In your precious tomorrow or the blessing of next Tuesday afternoon at work, there will come a time when someone or some situation shows you that some deep and profound spiritual change has already taken place. I don't know whether it will be a way to be of service or if it will be a way to connect. Perhaps it will be someone who challenges you. After all, the people who are hardest to love are the ones who need love the most, aren't they? Yes, you will notice this. I'm not sure if you'll notice a change in your words or your thoughts . . . or something profound in your heart or in your spirit. Something has already changed because you have remembered this forgotten part of yourself. Your true spiritual essence . . . with your unique set of gifts that have been given to you for a reason. Your destiny. Your reason for being here on this material plane . . . this planet. Some part of you knew that all along, didn't you?

Now I invite you to send this serenity, faith, and wisdom down into a button on your dominant index finger. Whenever you need a dose of this peace and purpose, all you need to do is press this button with your thumb. I wonder if you'll even feel that white spiritual light beginning to fill you up. And now gather any residual fear or resentment—visualizing it now as you blow it all into a balloon tied to your nondominant index finger. Now untie that balloon with your thumb . . . and watch as it floats far, far away. Can you see it becoming small?

And now those clouds are going to lift you back up . . . taking you back to the everyday world. In just a moment, become more alert as they lift you up . . . and by the time you reach the number one, you'll be fully awake, ready to take this peaceful, awake self into the world . . . to fill the world with your unique gifts . . .

12 . . . 11 . . . 10 . . . Those clouds lifting you back up, making you more alert . . .

9 . . . 8 . . . 7 . . . Those clouds bringing you up as you wiggle your fingers and toes . . .

6 . . . 5 . . . 4 . . . Becoming more and more alert now . . .

3 . . . 2 . . . 1 . . . Eyes open. Awake and alert. Ready to fill the world with the love of your precious spirit.

APPENDIX D

SVT Downloads

Thank you for purchasing *Your Subconscious Brain Can Change Your Life* by Dr. Mike Dow. This product includes free downloads. To access this bonus content, please visit www.hayhouse.com /download and enter the Product ID and Download Code as they appear below.

> *Product ID: 5854*
> *Download Code: Audio*

For further assistance, please contact Hay House Customer Care by phone—US (800) 654-5126 or INTL. CC+1760431-7695 —or by visiting www.hayhouse.com/contact.

Thank you again for your Hay House purchase. Enjoy!
Hay House, Inc. * P.O. Box 5100 * Carlsbad, CA 92018 * (800) 654-5126

Your Subconscious Brain Can Change Your Life Audio Download Track List

The 3/12/7 Method
SVT for Letting Go
SVT to Stress Less & Conquer Fears
SVT for Boosting Mood
SVT for Habits & Healthier Living
SVT for Bodily Healing
SVT for Sleep, Insomnia & Induced Dreaming
SVT to Boost Your Success
SVT to Deepen Your Spiritual Practice

Caution: This audio program features meditation/visualization exercises that render it inappropriate for use while driving or operating heavy machinery.

Publisher's note: Hay House products are intended to be powerful, inspirational, and life-changing tools for personal growth and healing. They are not intended as a substitute for medical care. Please use this audio program under the supervision of your care provider. Neither the author nor Hay House, Inc., assumes any responsibility for your improper use of this product.

ENDNOTES

Introduction

1. C.P. Le et al., "Chronic Stress in Mice Remodels Lymph Vasculature to Promote Tumour Cell Dissemination," *Nature Communications* 7, no. 10634 (March 2016), www.nature.com/articles/ncomms10634.

Chapter 1

1. English: Oxford Living Dictionaries, s.v. "subconscious," accessed April 30, 2018, https://en.oxforddictionaries.com/definition/subconscious.

2. Collins, s.v. "subconscious," accessed April 30, 2018, https://www .collinsdictionary.com/us/dictionary/english/subconscious.

3. G. Carli, "Animal Hypnosis and Pain," in *Hypnosis at its Bicentennial*, eds. F.H. Frankel and H.S. Zamansky (Boston: Springer, 1978): 69–77.

4. J.E.G. Charlesworth et al., "Effects of Placebos without Deception Compared with No Treatment: Protocol for a Systematic Review and Meta-Analysis," *Journal of Evidence-Based Medicine* 10, no. 2 (May 2017), https://doi .org/10.1111/jebm.12251.

5. T.F. Cohen, "The Power of Drug Color," *The Atlantic* (Oct. 14, 2014), www .theatlantic.com/health/archive/2014/10/the-power-of-drug-color/381156/.

6. J. Moncrieff, S. Wessely, and R. Hardy, "Active Placebos Versus Antidepressants for Depression," *Cochrane Database of Systematic Reviews* 1, no. CD003012 (2004), https://doi.org/10.1002/14651858.CD003012.pub2.

7. S. Metering, D. Bernstein, and R.G. Ley, "Imagery, Cerebral Laterality, and the Healing Process: A Cautionary Note," in *Healing Images: The Role of Imagination in Health*, ed. A.A. Sheikh (Amityville, NY: Baywood Publishing Company, 2003): 72.

8. *Inception*, written and directed by Christopher Nolan (Burbank, CA: Warner Bros. Pictures, 2010).

9. T. Orlick, *Embracing Your Potential* (Champagne, IL: Human Kinetics, 1998), 70.

10. J. Haley, *Jay Haley on Milton Erickson*, (New York: Brunner Mazel, 1993): 1–3, 5; "Biography of Milton H. Erickson" The Milton H. Erickson Foundation, accessed May 30, 2018, www.erickson-foundation.org/biography/.

Chapter 2

1. H. Yan, "California Mass Kidnapping: After Being Buried Alive, Victims Relive Nightmare," CNN.com, Dec. 28, 2015, www.cnn.com/2015/11/19/us/rewind -chowchilla-school-bus-kidnapping/index.html; D. Hevesi, "Ed Ray, Bus Driver During Kidnapping, Dies at 91," *New York Times*, May 18, 2012, www .nytimes.com/2012/05/19/us/ed-ray-bus-driver-who-helped-save-kidnapped -children-dies-at-91.html; and R. Thomas, Jr., "William S. Kroger, 89, Pioneer in Use of Hypnosis Treatment," *New York Times*, 1995, https://www.nytimes .com/1995/12/07/us/william-s-kroger-89-pioneer-in-use-of-hypnosis-as-treat ment.html.

2. S. Blakeslee, "This Is Your Brain Under Hypnosis," *New York Times*, November 22, 2005, nytimes.com/2005/11/22/science/this-is-your-brain-under-hypnosis .html.

3. B. Carey, "Herbert Spiegel, Doctor Who Popularized Hypnosis, Dies at 95," *New York Times*, January 9, 2010, https://www.nytimes.com/2010/01/10/ health/10spiegel.html?ref=obituaries.

4. P. McCormick, "Doctors' View of Hypnotherapy," *Delta Democrat-Times*, January 19, 1977.

5. P. McCormick, "Hypnosis: Alternative to Pills/Scalpel," *Pacific Stars and Stripes*, January 6, 1981.

6. H. Jiang et al. "Brain activity and functional connectivity associated with hypnosis." *Cerebral cortex* 27, no. 8 (2017): 4083–93.

7. A. Raz, J. Fan, and M.I. Posner, "Hypnotic Suggestion Reduces Conflict in the Human Brain," *Proceedings of the National Academy of Sciences of the United States of America* 102, no. 28 (2005): 9978–83.

8. Blakeslee, "Brain Under Hypnosis."

9. S. Derbyshire et al., "Cerebral Activation During Hypnotically Induced and Imagined Pain," *Neuroimage* 23, no. 1 (2004): 392–401.

10. Ibid.

11. M.P. Jensen, "The Neurophysiology of Pain Perception and Hypnotic Analgesia: Implications for Clinical Practice," *American Journal of Clinical Hypnosis* 51, no. 2 (2008): 123–148.

12. M.E. Faymonville et al., "Increased Cerebral Functional Connectivity Underlying the Antinociceptive Effects of Hypnosis," *Cognitive Brain Research* 17 (March 2003): 255–62.

13. P.W. Halligan et al., "Imaging Hypnotic Paralysis: Implications for Conversion Hysteria," *The Lancet* 355, no. 9208 (March 18, 2000): 986–87.

14. D. Oakley et al., "Hypnotic Imagery as a Treatment for Phantom Limb Pain: Two Case Reports and a Review," *Clinical Rehabilitation* 16, no. 4 (June 2002), 368–77.

15. S.J. Blakemore, D.A. Oakley, and C.D. Frith, "Delusions of Alien Control in the Normal Brain," *Neuropsychologia* 41, no. 8 (2003): 1058-67.

16. S. Kosslyn et al., "Hypnotic Visual Illusion Alters Color Processing in the Brain," *American Journal of Psychiatry* 157, no. 8 (August 2000): 1279–84.

17. P. Rainville et al., "Hypnosis Modulates Activity in Brain Structures Involved in the Regulation of Consciousness," *Journal of Cognitive Neuroscience* 14, no. 6 (2002): 887–901.

18. S. Bacon et al., "The Impact of Mood and Anxiety Disorders on Incident Hypertension at One Year," *International Journal of Hypertension* 2014, no. 953094 (2014).

19. J.W. Smoller et al., "Panic Attacks and Risk of Incident Cardiovascular Events among Postmenopausal Women in the Women's Health Initiative Observational Study," *Archives of General Psychiatry* 64, no. 10 (October 2007): 1153–60.

20. R. Kessler et al., "Insomnia and the Performance of US Workers: Results from the America Insomnia Survey," *Sleep* 34, no. 9 (September 2011): 1161–71.

21. J.D. Williams and J.H. Gruzelier, "Differentiation of Hypnosis and Relaxation by Analysis of Narrow Band Theta and Alpha Frequencies," *International Journal of Clinical and Experimental Hypnosis* 49, no. 3 (2001): 185–206.

22. N. Jokić-Begić and D. Begić, "Quantitative Electroencephalogram (qEEG) in Combat Veterans with Post-Traumatic Stress Disorder (PTSD)," *Nordic Journal of Psychiatry* 57, no. 5 (2003): 351–55.

23. A. Chen, "New Perspectives in EEG/MEG Brain Mapping and PET/fMRI Neuroimaging of Human Pain," *International Journal of Psychophysiology* 42, no. 2 (2001): 147–59.

24. Y.O. Fokina, A.M. Kulichenko, and V.B. Pavlenko, "Changes in the Power Levels of Cortical EEG Rhythms in Cats during Training Using Acoustic Feedback Signals," *Neuroscience and Behavioral Physiology* 40, no. 9 (Nov 2010): 951–54.

25. G. Buzsáki, *Rhythms of the Brain* (New York: Oxford University Press, 2006).

26. B.A. van der Kolk et al., "A Randomized Controlled Study of Neurofeedback for Chronic PTSD," *PLOS ONE* 11, no. 12 (December 2016): e0166752, https://doi.org/10.1371/journal.pone.0166752.

27. E.G. Peniston and P.J. Kulkosky, "α-θ-Brainwave Training and β-Endorphin Levels in Alcoholics," *Alcoholism: Clinical and Experimental Research* 13, no. 2 (1989): 271–79.

28. W.C. Scott et al., "Effects of an EEG Biofeedback Protocol on a Mixed Substance Abusing Population," *The American Journal of Drug and Alcohol Abuse* 31, no. 3 (2005): 455–69.

29. I. Lerner et al., "Baseline Levels of Rapid Eye Movement Sleep May Protect against Excessive Activity in Fear-Related Neural Circuitry," *Journal of Neuroscience* 37, no. 46 (November 2017): 11233–44.

30. Lerner et al., "Baseline Levels of Rapid Eye Movement," 11233–44; and A. Macmillan, "Why Dreaming May Be Important for Your Health," *TIME,* October 27, 2018, http://time.com/4970767/rem-sleep-dreams-health.

Chapter 3

1. I. Kirsch et al., "Hypnosis as an Adjunct to Cognitive-Behavioral Psychotherapy: A Meta-Analysis," *Journal of Consulting and Clinical Psychology* 63, no. 2 (1995): 214–19.

2. J. Kihlstrom, "Neuro-hypnotism: Prospects for Hypnosis and Neuroscience," *Cortex* 49, no. 2 (February 2013): 365–74; C. MacLeod-Morgan and L. Lack, "Hemispheric Specificity: A Physiological Concomitant of Hypnotizability," *Psychophysiology* 19, no. 6 (November 1982): 687–90; W.E. Edmonston and H.C. Moscovitz, "Hypnosis and Lateralized Brain Functions," *International Journal of Clinical Experimental Hypnosis* 38, no. 1 (January 1990): 70–84.

Chapter 4

1. I first learned about concepts similar to those I use in The 3/12/7 Method from Don E. Gibbons's book *Applied Hypnosis and Hyperempiria* (Bloomington, IN: iUniverse, 2000).

2. R. Naiman, "Dreamless: The Silent Epidemic of REM Sleep Loss," *Annals of the New York Academy of Sciences* 1406, no. 1 (2017): 77–85.

3. Ibid.

Chapter 6

1. W.S. Kroger and S.A. Schneider, "An Electronic Aid for Hypnotic Induction: A Preliminary Report," *International Journal of Clinical and Experimental Hypnosis* 7, no. 2 (1959): 93–98.

2. "FDA Drug Safety Communication: FDA Strengthens Warning That Non-aspirin Nonsteroidal Anti-inflammatory Drugs (NSAIDs) Can Cause Heart Attacks or Strokes," U.S. Food & Drug Administration, July 9, 2015, https://www.fda.gov/Drugs/DrugSafety/ucm451800.htm.

3. Jokić-Begić and D. Begić, "Quantitative Electroencephalogram (qEEG)," 351–55.

4. B. Bromm and J. Lorenz, "Neurophysiological Evaluation of Pain," *Electroencephalography and Clinical Neurophysiology* 107, no. 4 (1998): 227–53; and Chen, "New Perspectives," 147–59.

5. R. Lowes, "First Brain-Wave Test for ADHD Approved by FDA," *Medscape*, July 15, 2013, https://www.medscape.com/viewarticle/807869.

6. M. Joyce and D. Siever, "Audio-Visual Entrainment Program as a Treatment for Behavior Disorders in a School Setting," *Journal of Neurotherapy* 4, no. 2 (2000): 9–25.

7. J.A. Frederick et al., "EEG Coherence Effects of Audio-Visual Stimulation (AVS) at Dominant and Twice Dominant Alpha Frequency," *Journal of Neurotherapy* 8, no. 4 (2005): 25–42.

Chapter 7

1. U. Rutishauser et al., "Human Memory Strength Is Predicted by Theta-Frequency Phase-Locking of Single Neurons," *Nature* 464 (April 2010): 903–7; and M.E. Hasselmo, "What Is the Function of Hippocampal Theta Rhythm?—Linking Behavioral Data to Phasic Properties of Field Potential and Unit Recording Data," *Hippocampus* (September 12, 2005): 936–49.

2. D. Begić et al., "Electroencephalographic Comparison of Veterans with Combat-Related Post-traumatic Stress Disorder and Healthy Subjects," *International Journal of Psychophysiology* 40, no. 2 (April 2001): 167–72.

3. I'd often used Dr. Spiegel's method (Herbert & David Spiegel's book *Trance & Treatment* [American Psychiatric Publishing, 2008]) for hypnosis with my patients, and I realized they spontaneously fluttered their eyes side to side— that was my "aha" moment about bilateral stimulation. I also formally trained in accelerated resolution therapy, which uses bilateral stimulation.

4. J.D. Bremner, "Functional Neuroimaging in Post-traumatic Stress Disorder," *Expert Review of Neurotherapeutics* 7, no. 4 (April 1, 2007): 393–405.

5. M. Pagani et al., "Neurobiological Correlates of EMDR Monitoring—An EEG Study," *PLOS One* 7, no. 9 (2012): e45753.

6. E. Cardeña, "Hypnosis in the Treatment of Trauma: A Promising, but Not Fully Supported, Efficacious Intervention," *International Journal of Clinical and Experimental Hypnosis* 48, no. 2 (2000): 225–38.

7. Pagani et al., "Neurobiological Correlates," e45753.

8. The split screen concept originated with the Spiegels' book *Trance & Treatment* (American Psychiatric Publishing, 2008).

Chapter 8

1. E. Flammer, "Die Wirksamkeit von Hypnotherapie bei Angststörungen," *Hypnose—Zeitschrift für Hypnose und Hypnotherapie* 1, no. 1 (2006): 2.

2. R.A. Bryant et al., "The Additive Benefit of Hypnosis and Cognitive-Behavioral Therapy in Treating Acute Stress Disorder," *Journal of Consulting and Clinical Psychology* 73, no. 2 (2005): 334.

3. Kirsch et al., "Hypnosis as an Adjunct," 214.

4. Blakeslee, "Brain Under Hypnosis."

5. Raz, Fan, and Posner, "Hypnotic Suggestion Reduces Conflict," 9978–83.

6. B. Dias and K. Ressler, "Parental Olfactory Experience Influences Behavior and Neural Structure in Subsequent Generations," *Nature Neuroscience* 17 (2014): 89–96.

Chapter 9

1. A. Alladin and A. Alibhai, "Cognitive Hypnotherapy for Depression: An Empirical Investigation," *International Journal of Clinical and Experimental Hypnosis* 55, no. 2 (2007): 147–66.

2. M. Babyak et al., "Exercise Treatment for Major Depression: Maintenance of Therapeutic Benefit at 10 Months," *Psychosomatic Medicine* 62, no. 5 (2000): 633–38.

Chapter 10

1. G. Elkins et al., "Intensive Hypnotherapy for Smoking Cessation: A Prospective Study," *International Journal of Clinical and Experimental Hypnosis* 54, no. 3 (2006): 303–15.

2. T.P. Carmody et al., "Hypnosis for Smoking Cessation: A Randomized Trial," *Nicotine & Tobacco Research* 10, no. 5 (2008): 811–18.

3. I. Kirsch, "Hypnotic Enhancement of Cognitive-Behavioral Weight Loss Treatments: Another Meta-reanalysis," *Journal of Consulting and Clinical Psychology* 64, no. 3 (1996): 517.

4. R.J. Pekala et al., "Self-Hypnosis Relapse Prevention Training with Chronic Drug/Alcohol Users: Effects on Self-Esteem, Affect, and Relapse," *American Journal of Clinical Hypnosis* 46, no. 4 (Sept. 2011): 281–97.

5. D. Gibbons, *Applied Hypnosis and Hyperempiria* (Bloomington, IN: iUniverse, 2000).

6. M. Koivisto et al., "A Preconscious Neural Mechanism of Hypnotically Altered Colors: A Double Case Study," *PLOS ONE* 8, no. 8 (2013): e70900.

Chapter 11

1. Blakeslee, "Brain Under Hypnosis."

2. B. Enqvist et al., "Pre- and Perioperative Suggestion in Maxillofacial Surgery: Effects on Blood Loss and Recovery," *International Journal of Clinical and Experimental Hypnosis* 43, no. 3 (1995): 284–94.

3. C. Ginandes et al., "Can Medical Hypnosis Accelerate Post-surgical Wound Healing? Results of a Clinical Trial," *American Journal of Clinical Hypnosis* 45, no. 4 (2003): 333–51.

4. G.H. Montgomery et al., "Hypnosis for Cancer Care: Over 200 Years Young," *CA: A Cancer Journal for Clinicians* 63, no. 1 (2013): 31–44.

5. M. Faymonville et al., "Hypnosedation: A Valuable Alternative to Traditional Anaesthetic Techniques," *Acta Chirurgica Belgica* 99, no. 4 (1999): 141–46.

6. C. DeMarco, "Hypnosedation: Is It Possible to Have Surgery without General Anesthesia?" MD Anderson Cancer Center, July 13, 2017, https://www.md anderson.org/publications/cancerwise/2017/07/hypnosedation--surgery-with out-general-anesthesia.html.

7. M. Shah et al., "The Effect of Hypnosis on Dysmenorrhea," *International Journal of Clinical and Experimental Hypnosis* 62, no. 2 (2014): 164–78.

8. R. Beever, "The Effects of Repeated Thermal Therapy on Quality of Life in Patients with Type II Diabetes Mellitus," *The Journal of Alternative and Complementary Medicine* 16, no. 6 (2010): 677–81.

9. F. Oosterveld et al., "Infrared Sauna in Patients with Rheumatoid Arthritis and Ankylosing Spondylitis," *Clinical Rheumatology* 28, no. 1 (2009): 29.

10. "Autoimmune Diseases," National Institute of Environmental Health Sciences, July 16, 2018, https://niehs.nih.gov/health/topics/conditions/autoimmune/index.cfm.

11. L.S. Marchand et al., "Mesothelial Cell and Anti-nuclear Autoantibodies Associated with Pleural Abnormalities in an Asbestos Exposed Population of Libby MT," *Toxicology Letters* 208, no. 2 (2012): 168–73.

12. J.F. Nyland et al., "Fetal and Maternal Immune Responses to Methylmercury Exposure: A Cross-Sectional Study," *Environmental Research* 111, no. 4 (2011): 584–89.

13. R.J. Booth and K.R. Ashbridge, "A Fresh Look at the Relationship between the Psyche and Immune System: Teleological Coherence and Harmony of Purpose," *Advances* 9, no. 2 (1993): 4–23.

14. M.S. Torem, "Mind-Body Hypnotic Imagery in the Treatment of Auto-immune Disorders," *American Journal of Clinical Hypnosis* 50, no. 2 (2007): 157–70.

15. R.K. Naviaux et al., "Metabolic Features of Chronic Fatigue Syndrome," *Proceedings of the National Academy of Sciences* 113, no. 37 (2016): E5472–80.

16. J.K. Kiecolt-Glaser et al., "Hypnosis as a Modulator of Cellular Immune Dysregulation During Acute Stress," *Journal of Consulting and Clinical Psychology* 69, no. 4 (2001): 674.

17. N.P. Spanos et al., "Effects of Hypnotic, Placebo, and Salicylic Acid Treatments on Wart Regression," *Psychosomatic Medicine* 52, no. 1 (1990): 109–14.

18. J.D. Hamilton et al., "Dupilumab Improves the Molecular Signature in Skin of Patients with Moderate-to-Severe Atopic Dermatitis," *Journal of Allergy and Clinical Immunology* 134, no. 6 (2014): 1293–1300.

19. T.M. Laidlaw et al., "Reduction in Skin Reactions to Histamine After a Hypnotic Procedure," *Psychosomatic Medicine* 58, no. 3 (1996): 242–48.

20. J.R. Horton-hausknecht et al., "The Effect of Hypnosis Therapy on the Symptoms and Disease Activity in Rheumatoid Arthritis," *Psychology & Health* 14, no. 6 (2000): 1089–1104.

21. V.H. Gregg, "Hypnosis in Chronic Fatigue Syndrome," *Journal of the Royal Society of Medicine* 90, no. 12 (Dec. 1997): 682–83.

22. S. Noal et al., "One-Year Longitudinal Study of Fatigue, Cognitive Functions, and Quality of Life After Adjuvant Radiotherapy for Breast Cancer," *International Journal of Radiation Oncology* 81, no. 3 (2011): 795–803.

23. G.H. Montgomery et al., "Randomized Controlled Trial of a Cognitive-Behavioral Therapy Plus Hypnosis Intervention to Control Fatigue in Patients Undergoing Radiotherapy for Breast Cancer," *Journal of Clinical Oncology* 32, no. 6 (2014): 557.

24. A.V. Apkarian et al., "Pain and the Brain: Specificity and Plasticity of the Brain in Clinical Chronic Pain," *Pain* 152, no. 3 (2011): S49–64.

25. YaleNews, "Yale Study Shows Electrical Fields Influence Brain Activity," Yale University, July 14, 2010, https://news.yale.edu/2010/07/14/yale-study-shows-electrical-fields-influence-brain-activity.

26. Bromm and Lorenz, "Neurophysiological Evaluation of Pain," 227–53.

27. M.P. Jensen et al., "Effects of Non-pharmacological Pain Treatments on Brain States," *Clinical Neurophysiology* 124, no. 10 (2013): 2016–24.

28. M. Loggia et al., "Evidence for Brain Glial Activation in Chronic Pain Patients," *Brain* 138, no. 3 (2015): 604–15.

29. A. Koob, "The Root of Thought: What Do Glial Cells Do?" *Scientific American*, Oct. 27, 2009, https://www.scientificamerican.com/article/the-root-of-thought-what/.

30. D.R. Patterson et al., "Virtual Reality Hypnosis for Pain Associated with Recovery from Physical Trauma," *International Journal of Clinical and Experimental Hypnosis* 58, no. 3 (2010): 288–300.

31. D.R. Patterson et al., "Hypnosis Delivered through Immersive Virtual Reality for Burn Pain: A Clinical Case Series," *International Journal of Clinical and Experimental Hypnosis* 54, no. 2 (2006): 130–42.

32. M.P. Jensen et al., "Hypnotic Analgesia for Chronic Pain in Persons with Disabilities: A Case Series Abstract," *International Journal of Clinical and Experimental Hypnosis* 53, no. 2 (2005): 198–228.

33. M.P. Jensen et al., "Satisfaction with, and the Beneficial Side Effects of, Hypnotic Analgesia," *International Journal of Clinical and Experimental Hypnosis* 54, no. 4 (2006): 432–47.

34. M.P. Jensen et al., "Effects of Self-Hypnosis Training and EMG Biofeedback Relaxation Training on Chronic Pain in Persons with Spinal-Cord Injury," *International Journal of Clinical and Experimental Hypnosis* 57, no. 3 (2009): 239–68; M.P. Jensen et al., "A Comparison of Self-Hypnosis Versus Progressive Muscle Relaxation in Patients with Multiple Sclerosis and Chronic Pain," *International Journal of Clinical and Experimental Hypnosis* 57, no. 2 (2009): 198–221.

35. R.M. Lovell and A.C. Ford, "Global Prevalence of and Risk Factors for Irritable Bowel Syndrome: A Meta-analysis," *Clinical Gastroenterology and Hepatology* 10, no. 7 (2012): 712–21.

36. O. Palsson, "Hypnosis Treatment of Gastrointestinal Disorders: A Comprehensive Review of the Empirical Evidence," *American Journal of Clinical Hypnosis* 58, no. 2 (2015): 134–58.

37. O. Palsson, "Irritable Bowel," *Handbook of Medical and Psychological Hypnosis: Foundations, Applications, and Professional Issues,* ed. G. Elkins (New York: Springer Publishing Company, 2016): 285–289.

38. P. Lindfors et al., "Effects of Gut-Directed Hypnotherapy on IBS in Different Clinical Settings—Results from Two Randomized, Controlled Trials," *The American Journal of Gastroenterology* 107, no. 2 (2012): 276.

39. A.M. Vlieger et al., "Hypnotherapy for Children with Functional Abdominal Pain or Irritable Bowel Syndrome: A Randomized Controlled Trial," *Gastroenterology* 133, no. 5 (2007): 1430–36.

40. S. Banerjee et al., "Hypnosis and Self-Hypnosis in the Management of Nocturnal Enuresis: A Comparative Study with Imipramine Therapy," *American Journal of Clinical Hypnosis* 36, no. 2 (1993): 113–19.

41. J. Miller and E. Hoffman, "The Causes and Consequences of Overactive Bladder," *Journal of Women's Health* 15, no. 3 (2006): 251–60.

42. R. Doggweiler, "Hypnotherapy as a Complementary Treatment of Chronic Pelvic Pain Syndrome," International Continence Society, accessed July 23, 2018, https://www.ics.org/Abstracts/Publish/44/000237.pdf; and D.J. Carrico et al., "Guided Imagery for Women with Interstitial Cystitis: Results of a Prospective, Randomized Controlled Pilot Study," *The Journal of Alternative and Complementary Medicine* 14, no. 1 (2008): 53–60.

43. Carrico et al., "Guided Imagery for Women," 53–60.

44. Y.M. Komesu et al., "Hypnotherapy for Treatment of Overactive Bladder: An RCT Pilot Study," *Female Pelvic Medicine & Reconstructive Surgery* 17, no. 6 (2011): 308.

45. S. Aydin et al., "Efficacy of Testosterone, Trazodone and Hypnotic Suggestion in the Treatment of Non-organic Male Sexual Dysfunction," *British Journal of Urology* 77, no. 2 (1996): 256–60.

46. E.L. Calvert et al., "Long-Term Improvement in Functional Dyspepsia Using Hypnotherapy," *Gastroenterology* 123, no. 6 (2002): 1778–85.

47. G. Chiarioni et al., "Prokinetic Effect of Gut-Oriented Hypnosis on Gastric Emptying," *Alimentary Pharmacology & Therapeutics* 23, no. 8 (2006): 1241–49.

48. L. Keefer et al., "Gut-Directed Hypnotherapy Significantly Augments Clinical Remission in Quiescent Ulcerative Colitis," *Alimentary Pharmacology & Therapeutics* 38, no. 7 (2013): 761–71.

49. R.D. Anbar, "Self-Hypnosis for Patients with Cystic Fibrosis," *Pediatric Pulmonology* 30, no. 6 (2000): 461–65.

Appendix A

1. L. Xie et al., "Sleep Drives Metabolite Clearance from the Adult Brain," *Science* 342, no. 6156 (October 18, 2013): 373–77.

2. J.E. Kang et al., "Amyloid-Aβ Dynamics Are Regulated by Orexin and the Sleep-Wake Cycle," *Science* 326, no. 5955 (November 13, 2009): 1005–7.

3. M. Bellesi et al., "Effects of Sleep and Wake on Oligodendrocytes and Their Precursors," *The Journal of Neuroscience* 33, no. 36 (Sept. 4, 2013): 14288–300.

4. A. Qaseem et al., "Management of Chronic Insomnia Disorder in Adults: A Clinical Practice Guideline from the American College of Physicians," *Annals of Internal Medicine* 165, no. 2 (July 2016): 125–33.

5. R. Naiman, "Dreamless: The Silent Epidemic of REM Sleep Loss," *Annals of the New York Academy of Sciences* 1406, no. 1 (Aug. 15, 2017): 77–85.

6. D.L. Schacter, "EEG Theta Waves and Psychological Phenomena: A Review and Analysis," *Biological Psychology* 5, no. 1 (1977): 47–82.

7. Lerner et al., "Baseline Levels of Rapid Eye Movement," 11233–44.

8. M.J. Cordi, A.A. Schlarb, and B. Rasch, "Deepening Sleep by Hypnotic Suggestion," *Sleep* 37, no. 6 (June 1, 2014): 1143–52.

9. Ibid.

INDEX

A

Abundance, creating, xvi–xvii
Activating Subconscious Brain (Step 2),
    51–63
    brain mechanics for, 51–52
    deactivating subconscious and, 62
    re-alert following SVT, 62–63
    3/12/7 Method, 52–61
Adderall, 79
ADHD, 78–79
Alcoholism. See also Habit change and
    healthier living
    combination therapy for, 165–166
    SVT for, 38
Alertness
    AVE for, 77
    optional re-alert script (Step 2),
      overview, 62–63
    re-alert following SVT practices,
      108–109, 134–135, 159, 182,
      220–221
Alpha brain waves
    AVE for, 77
    meditation and, 53
    overview, 31–34
Amen, Daniel, 34–36
American Journal of Gastroenterology,
    The, 202
American Society of Clinical Hypnosis
    (ASCH), 15
Amygdala, 39, 113–116
Anesthesia, SVT vs./with, 185
Anterior cingulate cortex, 26, 27, 52
Anxiety. See Stress and fear, conquering
Audio tracks
    for letting go, 91–93
    3/12/7 Method, 63
    using scripts and, xxi
Audio-visual entrainment (AVE), 73–85
    advantages of, 76–78, 80–82
    cautions about, 78–80
    devices for, 73, 75–76, 82
    for elusive conditions, 187
    examples on drmikedow.com, 73,
      144
    history of, 73–74
    as interval training for brain, 83–84
    for pain, 74–75
    power of, 18
    synchronization with, 75–76
    3/12/7 Method vs., 80, 81
Autoimmune conditions, SVT for,
    188–192

B

Basal ganglia, 35
Baumann, Alex, 15
Bed-wetting, SVT for, 204
Beta brain waves
    alertness and, 53
    AVE for, 77–80
    overview, 32, 36
    pain feedback loop and, 196–197
    speed of, 43–44
Bilateral stimulation, 91–93
Bipolar disorder, 80
Bladder/urinary problems, SVT for,
    203–205
Blakeslee, Sandra, 114
Braid, James, 24
Brain, defined, 7–8
Brain anatomy. See also Habit change
    and healthier living; Healing;
    Mood boosting; Stress and fear,
    conquering
    amygdala, 39, 113–116
    EEG (electroencephalogram), 194
    glial cells, 198
    hypnosis and, 24–27
    limbic-hypothalamic-pituitary path-
      way, 188
    neurotransmitters (feel-good chemi-
      cals of brain), 112, 143–144, 162,
      164
    rest and effect on, 39
    right and left hemispheres, 43–44,
      91–93

Stroop test and, 25
SVT and scans of, 34–36
Brain Fog Fix, The (Dow), 83, 224
Brain scans
    EEG, 31, 34–36, 79, 194
    hypnosis and, 24–29
    SPECT, 34–36
Brain waves
    alpha brain waves, 31–34, 53, 77
    beta brain waves, 32, 36, 43–44, 53,
        77–80, 196–197
    delta brain waves, 33, 77, 223
    gamma brain waves, 31, 37
    pain feedback loop and, 196–197
    sleep and, 223, 225–226
    speeding up and slowing down,
        43–44
    subconscious and slow brain waves,
        5, 33, 37
    theta brain waves, overview, xv,
        32–34, 36–39 (*See also* Theta
        brain waves)
Brain Wave Synchronizer, 74–76
Breathing, awareness of, 56, 57
Building Bridges (Step 7), 71–72
B vitamins, 164

C

Cancer, SVT for, 184–187, 192
Chochilla kidnapping case, 21–22
Chronic fatigue syndrome (CFS), 189,
    191–192
Chronic pain, 192–195
Cognitive behavioral therapy (CBT)
    for boosting mood, 140–143
    cognitive behavioral therapy for
        insomnia (CBT-I), 224–226
    cognitive rehearsal, 69–70
    in combination with SVT and hyp-
        nosis, 18, 165–166
    for conquering stress and fear,
        111–114
    treating phobias with, xvii
Collective unconscious, 67
Color
    seeing, SVT Step 2, 56
    Stroop test and, 26
Combination therapy. *See also* Cog-
        nitive behavioral therapy (CBT);
        Hypnosis; Subconscious Visualiza-
        tion Technique (SVT)

effectiveness of, 165–166
SVT used with medication, 18
Confirmation bias, 139–140
Conscious brain
    analysis by, 5
    SVT Step 1 and (*See* Conscious Start
        to Subconscious Healing (SVT
        Step 1))
    worry and, xvi
Conscious Start to Subconscious Heal-
        ing (SVT Step 1)
    changing mantra with, 47–49
    employing conscious brain in SVT,
        42–44
    for letting go, 95
    pitfall thought patterns, defined,
        44–47 (*See also* Pitfall thought
        patterns)
    subconscious vs., 41–42
Conversion hysteria, 28
Cortisol, 37
Creating the Future (Step 5), 69–70
Creativity, SVT for, 38

D

Daydreaming, 4–6
Delta brain waves
    AVE for, 77
    overview, 33
    sleep and, 223
Depression. *See* Mood boosting
Destressing. *See* Stress and fear,
    conquering
Diabetes, SVT for, 186
Dr. Oz Show, The, 11
Drmikedow.com (website)
    AVE examples, 73, 187
    on CBT-I, 226
    on conquering stress and phobias,
        113
    free downloads, 243–244
    on neurotransmitters and vitamins,
        144, 164
    SVT practices on, 232
Dopamine
    B vitamins for, 164
    mood and, 143–144
    sensation seeking and, 162
Dow, Mike
    The Brain Fog Fix, 83, 224

drmikedow.com (website), 73, 113,
144, 164, 187, 226, 243–244
Heal Your Drained Brain, 83, 113,
224–225
Dreaming, theta brain waves and, 39.
See also Sleep

E

Eczema, SVT for, 191
Edison, Thomas, 38
EEG (electroencephalogram)
ADHD diagnosis with, 79
function of, 31
pain relief and, 194
during SVT, 34–36
Elusive conditions, SVT for, 200–205
Emory University, 118
Enhancing the Present (Step 4), 68–69
Epigenetic inheritance, 118
Epilepsy, 80
Eternal Sunshine of the Spotless Mind
(film), 23
Exercise, for mood boost, 143–144

F

False memory cases (1990s), 22
Fear. *See* Stress and fear, conquering
Feedback loops
elusive conditions and, 201
pain and, 195–196
Fight-or-flight response, 76
Flight/freeze response, 189
Floating sensation, 61
FMRI (functional magnetic resonance
imaging), 26, 27, 31, 34
Food sensitivity, SVT for, 203
Freud, Sigmund, 67
Frontal lobe, 36
Functional abdominal pain (FAP), SVT
for, 202–203

G

GABA, 112, 143–144
Gamma brain waves, 31, 37
Genetics
elusive conditions and, 200–201
epigenetic inheritance, 118
genetic testing, 187
Glial cells, 198

Goals
achieving success with, 163,
231–235
focusing on, 163
for letting go, 87–88
positive visualization for, 30
setting goals with SVT, 14–15
SMART (specific, measurable,
achievable, relevant, time
sensitive) goals, 14

H

Habit change and healthier living,
161–182
benefits of SVT for, 165–166
changing senses for, 167–168
habit formation, 161–163
re-alert following SVT, 182
script for, 169–182
SVT frequency for, 168–169
understanding deficiencies in,
163–165
Hallucinations, creating, 29–30, 167–
168. *See also* Visualization
Healing, 183–221
boosting immunity for, 187–192
from "elusive conditions," 200–205
integrative visualization for,
186–187
mindbody connection for, 183–186
from pain, 192–200
re-alert following SVT, 220–221
script for, 206–220
SVT for bodily healing, 205–206
Heal Your Drained Brain (Dow), 83, 113,
224–225
HPV, 190–191
Hypnosis
alpha and theta brain waves
boosted by, 34
brain scans showing effects of,
24–27
Chochilla kidnapping case, 21–22
in combination with SVT and CBT,
18, 165–166
false memory cases (1990s), 22
hypnosedation, 185
Mesmer's work on, 24
mindbody connection and, 29–31,
183–186

for pain, 199
willingness for, 22–23

I

Ibuprofen, 185–186
Immune system
  autoimmune conditions, 188–192
  boosting, for healing, 187–192
  elusive conditions and, 200
  preautoimmunity, 188
  T cells and, xvi, 31
Inception (film), 12–14
Information processing/interpretation
  by subconscious, 3–4
  top-down processing and, 114–116
Insight, 66–67
Insomnia. *See* Sleep
Insula, 25–27, 52
Integrative visualization, 186–187
Irritable bowel syndrome (IBS)
  hypnosis for, 30
  SVT for, 200, 202–203

J

Jung, C., 67

K

Kroger, William, 73–74, 222

L

Lancet, The, 28
Learned Optimism (Seligman), 141
Left/right hemispheres of brain, 43–44,
  91–93
Legal issues, SVT cautions about, 17
Letting go, 87–109
  biology of SVT in, 91–93
  preparing for, 95–96
  re-alert following SVT, 108–109
  reasons for, 88–91
  regular practice of SVT for, 94
  script for, 93–108
  setting goals for SVT, 87–88
Light-sensitive migraine, 80
Limbic-hypothalamic-pituitary pathway, 188

M

Major dissociative disorders, SVT cautions about, 16
Mantra
  changing, 47–49

confirmation bias and, 139–140
McCormick, David, 195
MD Anderson, 185
Medication
  AVE vs., 74–75, 79, 81–82
  combination therapy of SVT and, 18
  for depression, 143–144
  healing with SVT vs., 184–186,
    190–194, 202
  placebos and, 9
  side effects of, 9–10
Memory
  accessing forgotten memories, xv
  AVE and, 79–80
  conquering fear and stress, 114–116
  happy memories, 90
  "recording" positive memories over
    negative memories, 23–24
  reprocessing negative memories,
    66–68, 89
  subconscious for discovering past,
    13–14
  suppression of, 89
Menstrual cramps, SVT for, 185–186
Mental health and mental illness. *See
  also* Mood boosting; Stress and
  fear, conquering
  glial cells and, 198
  Mesmer on, 24
  SVT cautions about, 16–17, 80, 140
  top-down processing for, 27
Mesmer, Franz, 24
Migraine, 80
Mind, brain vs., 7–8
Mindbody connection
  for healing, 183–186
  science of subconscious brain and,
    29–31
  SVT for, xv
Mindfulness
  Activating the Subconscious Brain
    (Step 2) for, 56
  defining mind vs. brain, 8
  Mindfulness-Based Cognitive Therapy (MBCT), 142–143 (*See also*
    Cognitive behavioral therapy
    (CBT))
Mood boosting, 137–159
  CBT with SVT for, 140–144
  medication for, 137–138
  re-alert following SVT, 159
  science of, 138–140
  SVT script for, 144–159

Music, theta brain waves and, 33

N

Negative emotion. *See* Positive vs. negative emotion
Neurotransmitters
  dopamine, 143, 162, 164
  GABA, 112, 143
  serotonin, 112, 143, 164
Nutrition
  power of, 18
  vitamins and, 164

O

Obesity, chronic pain and, 193–194
Occipital lobe, 36
Ohio State University, 31
Open-label placebos, 9
Oz, Dr., 11

P

Pain. *See also* Healing
  AVE for, 74–75
  chronic, 192–195
  as feedback loop, 195–198
  medication vs. SVT for, 193–194
  virtual reality (VR) for, 198–200
Painter, Kelly, 185
Paralysis by analysis (pitfall thought pattern)
  defined, 44–45
  habit formation and, 162–163
  letting go and, 92
Parasympathetic nervous system, 76
Parietal cortex, 25, 26
Permanence (pitfall thought pattern)
  defined, 45
  depression and, 141–142
  healing and, 197–198
Personalization (pitfall thought pattern)
  defined, 45
  depression and, 141–142
Personal unconscious, 67
Pervasiveness (pitfall thought pattern)
  defined, 45–46
  depression and, 141–142
Pessimism (pitfall thought pattern), 46
PET scans, 28
Phantom limb pain, 28

Phobias. *See* Stress and fear, conquering
Photosensitive epilepsy, 80
Physical health, SVT cautions about, 17
Pitfall thought patterns
  definitions, 44–47
  depression and, 141–142
  extinguishing, 68
  habit formation and, 162–163
  healing and, 197–198
  letting go and, 92
Placebos
  hypnosis compared to, 30
  open-label placebos, 9
Planting Positivity (Step 6), 70–71
Polarization (pitfall thought pattern), 46
Positive vs. negative emotion
  changing mantra and, 47–49
  Inception (film) on, 12–13
  Planting Positivity (Step 6), 70–71
  science of subconscious brain and memory, 23–24
  virtual reality treatment and, 199
Power of suggestion. *See* Suggestibility
Preautoimmunity, 188
Prefrontal cortex, 25–27, 35, 52, 194, 236
Psychic thinking (pitfall thought pattern), 46

R

Radar, brain's reaction to, 74
Rapid eye movement (REM), 39, 53, 225–226. *See also* Sleep
Raz, Amir, 25–26
Reprocessing, 66–68, 89
Rest. *See* Sleep
Rest-and-digest response, 76
Revising the Past (Step 3)
  bilateral stimulation with, 91–93
  overview, 66–67
Rheumatoid arthritis, SVT for, 186, 191
Right/left hemispheres of brain, 43–44, 91–93

S

Salicylic acid, 190–191
Schneider Instrument Company, 74
Science of subconscious brain, 21–39
  brain wave types, defined, 31–34,
    36–39 (*See also* Brain waves)
  Chochilla kidnapping case example,
    21–22
  EEG and SPECT, 34–36
  hypnosis and brain scans, 24–29
  hypnosis and willingness, 22–23
  mindbody connection and, 29–31
  positive vs. negative memory and,
    23–24
Scripts
  about bonus scripts, 18
  bonus material, 18
  for conquering stress and fear,
    120–134
  for habit change and healthier liv-
    ing, 169–182
  for healing, 206–220
  for letting go, 93–108
  for mood boost, 144–159
  optional re-alert scripts, 62–63 (*See
    also* Alertness)
  for sleep, insomnia and induced
    dreaming, 226–230
  for spirituality, 236–241
  for success, 231–235
  for 3/12/7 Method (SVT Step 2),
    55–61
Seligman, Martin, 141
Sensation seeking, 162
Serotonin
  B vitamins for, 164
  for conquering stress and fear, 112
  mood and, 143–144
Sexual function, SVT for, 205
Sleep
  AVE and, 77, 80
  conquering fear and stress for, 117
  insomnia and subconscious-domi-
    nant state, 7
  SVT for sleep, insomnia and
    induced dreaming, 223–230
SMART (specific, measurable, achievable, relevant, time sensitive)
  goals, 14

Sound, Activating the Subconscious
  Brain (Step 2) and, 56
SPECT (single-photon emission computed tomography) scans, 34–36
Spiegel, Herbert, 24–25
Spirituality
  Revising the Past (Step 3) for, 67
  script for, 236–241
  theta brain waves and, 87–88
Stress and fear, conquering, 111–135
  biology of, 113–116
  conquering with SVT, overview, 111
  Conscious Start to Subconscious
    Healing (Step 1) and, 120
  re-alert following SVT, 134–135
  script for, 120–134
  stress as cause of habits, 162
  suggestibility and, 116–119
  SVT preparation for conquering
    stress and fear, 119–120
  using feel-good brain chemicals for,
    112
  virtual reality treatment for phobias,
    199
Stroop test, 26
Subconscious, 3–19. *See also* Activating
  Subconscious Brain (Step 2); Science of subconscious brain
  activating, 8–10
  brain vs. mind, definitions, 7–8
  daydreaming with, 4–6
  defined, 6–7
  discovering past with, 13–14 (*See
    also* Memory)
  for empowerment, 16–18
  goal setting for future with, 14–15
  information processing by, 3–4
  positive vs. negative emotion and,
    12–13
  suggestibility and, 10–12, 17
  SVT program steps and, 18–19 (*See
    also* Subconscious Visualization
    Technique (SVT))
  theta brain waves as signature of, 36
Subconscious Visualization Technique
  (SVT)
  applications of (*See* Habit change
    and healthier living; Healing;
    Letting go; Mood boosting; Sleep;

Spirituality; Stress and fear, conquering; Success)
cautions about, 16–17, 78–80, 140
in combination with CBT and hypnosis, 18, 165–166
frequency of, 52–53, 65, 72, 94, 168
mini-practice, xviii–xx
power boosting (See Audio-visual entrainment (AVE))
program steps, overview, 18–19
Step 1 (Conscious Start to Subconscious Healing), 41–49
Step 2 (Activating Subconscious Brain), 51–63
Step 3 (Revising the Past), 66–67
Step 4 (Enhancing the Present), 68–69
Step 5 (Creating the Future), 69–70
Step 6 (Planting Positivity), 70–71
Step 7 (Building Bridges), 71–72
subconscious activation with, xiii–xviii
Substance abuse. See also Habit change and healthier living
combination therapy for, 165–166
SVT for, 38
Success, 163, 231–235
Suggestibility
conquering fear and stress with, 116–119
false memory cases (1990s), 22
power of, 10–12, 17
Superman (films), 112
Surgery, SVT for, 183–184
Sympathetic nervous system, 76
SVT. See Subconscious Visualization Technique (SVT)

T

T cells
activating immune system and, xvi
boosting, 31
Theta brain waves
for accessing forgotten memories, xv
AVE for, 76–80
EEG of SVT process and, 36
functions of, 32–34, 36–38
pain feedback loop and, 197

REM sleep and dreaming, 39, 53
sleep and, 223, 225–226
speed of, 43–44
spirituality and, 87–88
3/12/7 Method (SVT Step 2 component). See also Activating Subconscious Brain (Step 2)
AVE vs., 80, 81
deactivating subconscious and optional re-alert script, 62–63
purpose of, 52–55
script for, 55–61
using audio track for, 53–54, 63
Titanic (film), 90–91
Top-down processing
changing, 26–27
habit formation and, 164–165
for interpreting information, 114–116

U

Unconscious, defined, 6–7
Urinary problems, SVT for, 203–205

V

Van der Kolk, Bessel, 113
Virtual reality (VR), 198–200
Visualization
choosing imagery for, 54
creating visual sensation (hallucination), 29–30, 167–168
effect on occipital lobes, 36
integrative visualization for healing, 186–187
12 floors relaxation exercise, 59, 62–63

W

White blood cells, 190

Z

Zoloft, 143–144

ABOUT THE AUTHOR

Dr. Mike Dow, Psy.D., Ph.D., is a *New York Times* best-selling author and has been called "America's go-to therapist." In addition to his private practice in Los Angeles, he has hosted shows on TLC, VH1, E!, Investigation Discovery, and Logo. He is part of Dr. Oz's core team of experts, a recurring guest cohost on *The Doctors*. Dr. Mike also makes regular appearances on *Today, Rachael Ray, Wendy Williams, Bethenny, Meredith Vieira, Ricki Lake, Nancy Grace,* and *Dr. Drew on Call*. He is a member of the American Society for Clinical Hypnosis and the Society for Clinical and Experimental Hypnosis. Dr. Mike is a graduate of USC where he was a Presidential Scholar. Learn more at drmikedow.com.

Hay House Titles of Related Interest

YOU CAN HEAL YOUR LIFE, the movie, starring Louise Hay & Friends
(available as a 1-DVD program, an expanded 2-DVD set,
and an online streaming video)
Learn more at www.hayhouse.com/louise-movie

THE SHIFT, the movie,
starring Dr. Wayne W. Dyer
(available as a 1-DVD program, an expanded 2-DVD set,
and an online streaming video)
Learn more at www.hayhouse.com/the-shift-movie

***

THE BIOLOGY OF BELIEF: Unleashing the Power of Consciousness, Matter & Miracles, by Bruce H. Lipton, Ph.D.

CONTROL STRESS, by Paul McKenna, Ph.D.

RESILIENCE FROM THE HEART: The Power to Thrive in Life's Extremes, by Gregg Braden

SECRETS OF MEDITATION: A Practical Guide to Inner Peace and Personal Transformation, by davidji

YOU ARE THE PLACEBO: Making Your Mind Matter, by Dr. Joe Dispenza

All of the above are available at your local bookstore,
or may be ordered by contacting Hay House (see next page).

***

We hope you enjoyed this Hay House book. If you'd like to receive our online catalog featuring additional information on Hay House books and products, or if you'd like to find out more about the Hay Foundation, please contact:

Hay House, Inc., P.O. Box 5100, Carlsbad, CA 92018-5100
(760) 431-7695 or (800) 654-5126
(760) 431-6948 (fax) or (800) 650-5115 (fax)
www.hayhouse.com® • www.hayfoundation.org

———

Published in Australia by:
Hay House Australia Pty. Ltd., 18/36 Ralph St., Alexandria NSW 2015
Phone: 612-9669-4299 • *Fax:* 612-9669-4144 • www.hayhouse.com.au

Published in the United Kingdom by:
Hay House UK, Ltd., Astley House, 33 Notting Hill Gate, London W11 3JQ
Phone: 44-20-3675-2450 • *Fax:* 44-20 3675-2451 • www.hayhouse.co.uk

Published in India by: Hay House Publishers India,
Muskaan Complex, Plot No. 3, B-2, Vasant Kunj, New Delhi 110 070
Phone: 91-11-4176-1620 • *Fax:* 91-11-4176-1630 • www.hayhouse.co.in

———

Access New Knowledge.
Anytime. Anywhere.

Learn and evolve at your own pace
with the world's leading experts.

www.hayhouseU.com